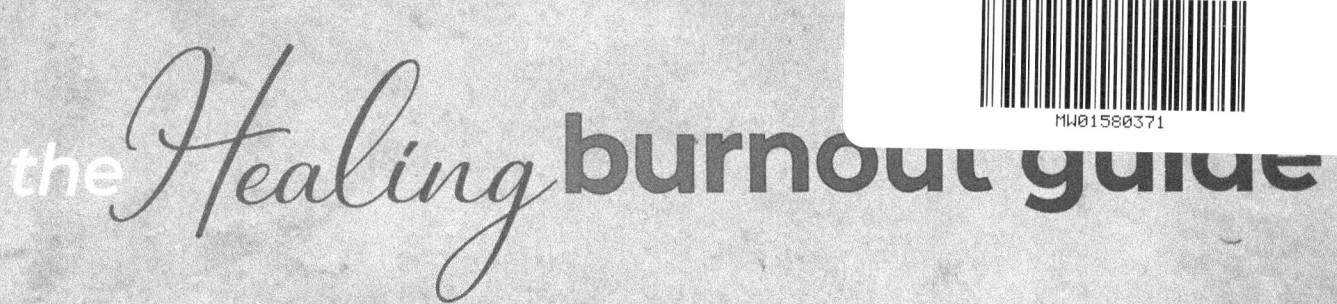

A collection of daily perspectives, reflection & artistry

Competent

Dr. Richard C. Scepura, DNP, MBA/MHA, RN, NEA-BC, CDN

curation by nancy nixon ensign

Copyright © 2021 Victorem Enterprises, LLC.

All Rights Reserved. This book contains material protected under International and Federal Copyright Laws and Treaties. Any unauthorized reprint or use of this material is prohibited. No part of this book may be reproduced or transmitted in any form or by any means, electronic or mechanical, including photocopying, recording, or by any information storage and retrieval system without express written permission from the author/publisher.

Hard Cover ISBN: 978-1-953806-75-8
Paperback ISBN: 978-1-953806-81-9
Journal (B&W) ISBN: 979-8-9851198-4-8
Journal (Color) ISBN:979-8-9851198-3-1
Workbook ISBN: 979-8-9851198-5-5
eBook ISBN: 979-8-9851198-2-4
Hybrid ISBN: 979-8-9851198-6-2

Disclaimer

Neither this nor any other book should be used as a substitute for professional medical care or treatment. It is advisable to seek the guidance of a healthcare provider before implementing any of the approaches to health suggested in this book. The book was written to provide select information to the public concerning burnout and related topics. Research in this field is ongoing and subject to interpretation. Neither the publisher, the producer, nor the author takes any responsibility for any possible consequences from any treatment, action, or application of medicine or preparation by any person reading or following the information in this book.

Dedication

For Lamby

This book was written with the memory of author, Col. Wm. Hunter, in mind. He wrote common sense inspirational books such as *Pep, Think, and Ginger Snaps* in the late 1910's when the Spanish Flu, Russian Revolution, and First World War were the backdrop. Remarkably, similar situations have occurred in 2020 with the Covid-19 Pandemic, Russian aggression with social media, and a divisive civil political landscape. *Think* was a thrift store find and was given to the author of this book as a gift decades ago. The author, Richard Scepura, acknowledges all the hard workers in the U.S.A. and other countries around the globe that may be feeling overworked, stressed, and effects of burnout. Through reading, reflecting, connecting with inspiring art, and journaling, the process of healing from burnout can begin.

Acknowledgements

This book was a labor of love and written during the last two semesters of my doctoral program while undergoing career transitioning during the coronavirus pandemic. Originally, it was a small seed idea that morphed into a more extensive project. My first thank you must be to heaven and my mother, father, and sister for the many years of nurturing and support given to me as the youngest child. The generous support of my loving father during coronavirus time period while writing this book was immense, and for that, I am forever grateful. My aunts & uncles, many cousins, and of course my doggies, *Hank, Veda, and Birdie*. I hope that I make my entire family proud in *all I do*. (I try- even though I can be a little rascal).

Next, I want to praise each and every artist who willingly volunteered to be part of this project, offering their labors of love in images for the benefit of many. If there is a particular piece that you have connected with, I hope you will find the artists' contact information in that section of the book and reach out to them to support, acknowledge, or show interest in their work. It is so important to offer recognition, and I am certain each would appreciate that very much. Their work inspired me a great deal while spending many hours researching and writing the book at the Patterson Library in Westfield, NY (*Chautauqua County*).

This brings me to a very special thank you to a dear friend of mine, Nancy Nixon Ensign, the Curator of *Octagon Gallery* and primary artist showcased in this book and covers. I have known her for over thirty years from our college days at *Rochester Institute of Technology* together. She'd offer me a lift home when needed and literally went the extra mile, beyond her own town, to make sure I got home safely. Well, after so much time of lives apart and away, reconnecting together on this project challenged us both! There were days we laughed, cried, shouted, pulled teeth, and leapt for joy. It was kismet when we each knew and agreed on an idea or work of art. Her keen curation skill made the process almost seem effortless in retrospect, and she still gives me a big heartfelt lift.

Once the art was situated, my attention became much more focused on refinement and much gratitude to our first contributing editor, Tiffany Smith. Tiffany and I spent some evenings (after already busy workdays) of a 4-month pleasant period, to ready the draft manuscripts. Without

Tiffany, the constant push and responsibility toward completing each season of the book might have been adrift. I am forever thankful for all her assistance and organizational skills, helping me keep versions of the draft manuscripts in order. I highly recommend Tiffany for your technical writing or editing needs. (See: www.tlynnseditingservice.net)

Next, how do you ever graciously thank your eighth-grade English teacher enough for volunteering during her busy schedule to read and peer-review your work so many years after graduating high school? With much gratitude, I thank Dr. Jane Blystone, Ph.D., MJE, who volunteers on the prestigious *Journalism Education Association, Inc.* (JEA) Scholastic Press Rights Committee, JEA Certification Committee, and is a JEA Mentor. I hope the book brought some joy and peace for you. After all these years, you are still mentoring me, and you are so appreciated. Thank you kindly for writing the Forward.

Another peer reviewer was the Director of my Nursing program at *Clarion and Edinboro Universities*, Dr. Meg Larson. Meg was my professor and committee chair for a completely different project during the doctoral studies, in addition to peer-reviewing this book. She is one of the most patient educators I know, and she steered me in the right direction (encouraging me to write and publish), and I am grateful to her as well. I appreciate her taking the time to digest the work, offer feedback and input. Her flexibility allowed me to challenge myself in new ways of thinking and growing. I hope she enjoyed the topics and art, as well and her time reading the book. In some small way, I hope it helped inspire her. I'm sure she had a giggle, grimace, or grin while reviewing! I thank her greatly for writing the additional Forward.

Next came the final review of the manuscript with contributing editor, Jessica Olma. Jessica came recommended to us by *Spotlight Publishing*. Jessica's editing refined the works to expand our audience. It took me a little while, but we reached the end of the final manuscript as I began writing these acknowledgments. I am forever grateful for her expertise, and professionalism. I hope the book brought insight and joy to her as well, and that the information in the book was of interest and helpful. Thank you for making the final editing phase very smooth, Jessica! Her business is at Scribe Syndicate, and I recommend her to all.

After I had the first round of peer reviewed manuscript completed, I invited other reviewers to read the books. I wanted to be certain that there was a multi-disciplinary review from professionals before going to print. Dr. Matthew Conner, MD, Dr. Deborah Cohan, MD, MPH, Dr. Preston Davis, PsyD, Josephine Poulin, MSN, APRN, FNP-C, and Dr. Patricia Boulogne, DC, CCSP, MaoM, AP, CFLP, CFMP. I am so thankful for their time, efforts, and appreciate their feedback. I also would like to thank Dr. Patricia Benner, Nurse Theorist and Author of *From Novice to Expert* for inspiring this work.

Our graphic designer for the second book in the series is Tom Olson, owner of Pixel-Pencil Studio. Tom really took the design of the second book in our series to an evolved level and we are very grateful for his expertise. Working with Tom is such a pleasure, he is organized, creative and very timely. I would highly recommend Tom and his business, which helps authors make their project come to life- Thank you, Tom!

Becky Norwood, wise and knowledgeable boutique publisher, can be found at Spotlight Publishing. Becky was recommended to me by Dr. Pat Boulogne, author of *Why are you Sick, Fat, and Tired?* (An Amazon #1 best seller). I highly recommend Dr. Pat's "Smarter than Medicine" program, as I was one of her clients recently, and her course is amazing, even life-changing! Find her at Health Team Network. Dr. Pat reached her number one status on Amazon because of the tireless support and talent of Becky and *Spotlight Publishing*. I recommend Spotlight Publishing for all your "authorpreneur needs." Let Becky show you how to do more than reach number one and be the best version of you.

With that, last but not least, are the many other friends, colleagues, and loved ones along the way in my life that have been supportive, not just during this period of creating the book, but faithfully through thick and thin. They know who they are: Doreen, Liza, Vicki, Mary Jane S., Audra, Nate, Alain, Mary Jo, Sharin, David, Jason, Douglas, Jimmy, Avi, Ian, my next-door neighbors Nicholas, Tiffany, and Rosie. Dawn and Nicholas & Brandon, Elizabeth G, Michael V., Nurse Joy, Heidi (my teacher of *Nadi Shodhana Pranayama*), Preston, Daphne, Maria, Phil, Libby O., the entire Boston *Eclipse* crew including Brenda, David, Cyndi, Bob, Steve, Paul, Marianne, Denise, Boston's North End *La Summa* Barbara and Siobhan from *Pomodoro*, through the years (forever grateful for beautiful memories), my North End friends David Archer, Billy, Desi, Chip, and hometown friends Lisa Conti, Julie & Randy (always missed), Lisa Monte, Ruthie and Jan, Toni & JT, Uncle Clay, the Clines, Dunster Street Pat and Scottie, my *Maui Ohana*- Kelly, Erina, Uncle Brett, Dale and April, my special JP 39-bus friend, Peeps, Dr. Paula Sperry (talk radio host at *WOMR Provincetown*), the countless friends and neighbors that inspired me over decades in Provincetown in the East End and West End, St. Elizabeth's, BIDMC, Mass General and Seattle Children's dialysis nurses, and countless others (those I may have missed acknowledging due to my humanness). To all my professors and *alma maters* RIT, UMASS Boston, Pfeiffer U., and Clarion and Edinboro Universities- *Thank you, thank you.*

Preface

Considerable improvements in clinical work and learning environments in every healthcare setting must be prioritized for all disciplines to prevent and mitigate clinician burnout and foster wellbeing for the overall health of medical professionals, patients, and the nation. According to *The National Academies of Sciences, Engineering, & Medicine* (2019), "between 35 and 54 percent of U.S. nurses and physicians experience burnout symptoms, along with 45 to 60 percent of medical students and residents." Many studies have indicated burnout to be a common problem among all clinical disciplines and across care settings.[1]

Studies conducted in 2020 have shown further evidence of the rising burnout. One study known as the *Physicians' Foundation/Merritt Hawkins Study* concluded that about 55 percent of healthcare workers described their job as negative due to the conditions. The *Medscape* study revealed that physician burnout has increased by 2 percent since 2018. *The AMN Healthcare* biennial nursing study revealed that a rising 63 percent of nurses reported burnout and 44 percent often wanted to quit as a result.[2]

Making matters even more serious, the start of 2020 introduced our world to the pandemic known as COVID-19 (coronavirus 2019), which no one was prepared to handle. Stress, anxiety, and burnout among healthcare workers during the outbreak reached an all-time high due to the fear of catching the virus and spreading it to others, as well as the uncertainty of how the outbreak would affect us overall both socially and economically. The only option for healthcare workers to make it through this time period is/was to remain hopeful and look for opportunities to practice self-care, professional advocacy, celebrate successes, and find time to take breaks from stress. It is imperative for employers to encourage their employees to practice acts of self-care in an attempt to reduce stress and burnout.[3] These are alarming statistics of burnout in healthcare workers. Imagine what other industries may have similar situations.

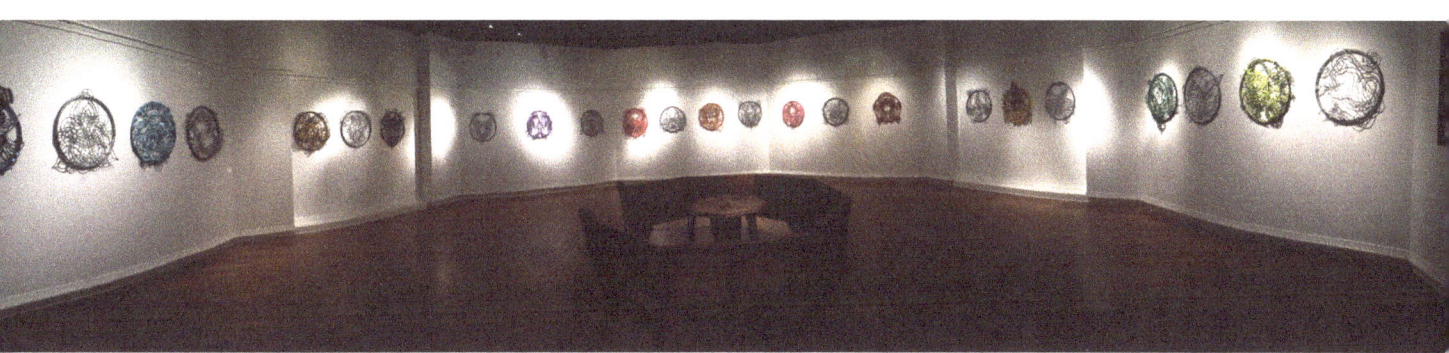

Jon Chisholm in Octagon Gallery

The Octagon Gallery is part of the world-famous Patterson Library in Westfield, NY (Chautauqua County) and hosts several artists for monthly exhibitions in a variety of mediums.

Foreword

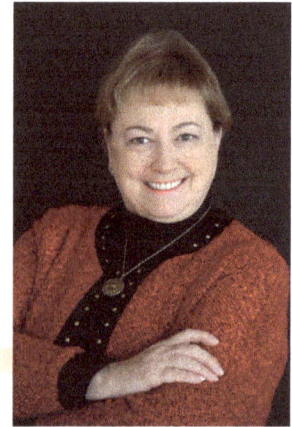

In a time of great stress for many, this pandemic has moved many professionals in healthcare, education, and other essential services into burnout mode. In this 365-day self-reflection journal Richard has prepared, the reader will practice strong reflective thinking that provides a researched approach to reduce stress, and concerning day-to-day frustrations that lead to burnout. Richard has always been an empathetic person. I first met him when he joined my yearbook staff in high school. As his teacher, I watched his great love for helping people. As he graduated and followed a career path in healthcare as a nurse, I was so impressed that he continued to be a helper and empathetic individual. His career has led him to be a traveling nurse, nurse manager, director, consultant, and continue his education at both the graduate and doctoral levels.

Richard has seen and helped deal with burnout in his profession. We have talked about this for some time and I am so pleased to see this book emerge as a tool for individuals who work with many patients, clients, students, customers on any given day to deal with the stress of caring for others. This reflection journal is the outworking of his skill in caring for other nurses, healthcare professionals, and the public. It is a much needed reflective tool for anyone in our time. Each season of this self-reflection journal gives the reader the option of reflecting in writing and/or in thoughtful self-reflection about ways to calm the mind and heart. The art he has selected also provides beautiful aesthetic experiences for the reader. Professionals who feel stationary in their careers will find this journal a perfect way to articulate goals for future advancement and to develop self-confidence.

It is my great pleasure to recommend this book to you as I have read every word and experienced the uplifting nature of these daily reflection exercises Richard has presented in this journaling workbook.

Enjoy,

Jane Blystone, PhD, MJE
JEA Mentor Program Chair
JEA Certification Committee
PA School Press Association Board of Directors

Foreword

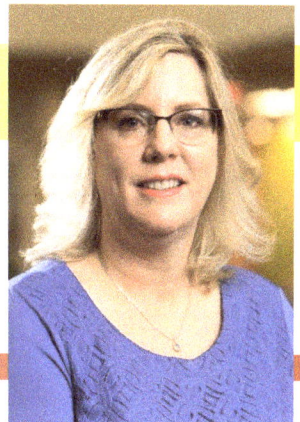

In living memory, there has never been a time WITH SO MANY EVENTS that have touched SO MANY PEOPLE across all walks of life. In normal times, professionals in some careers face high burnout rates. This is, of course, exacerbated by the global pandemic, which strains them professionally, and, in many cases, personally.

We all hope that we have a period of healing coming soon. The world's trauma is largely beyond any individual control, which can lead to increased feelings of pain, disempowerment, and burnout. This self-reflection journal is a wonderful resource that allows readers to spend as much or as little time as they have and still make an impact on their mental health and carry on in their essential careers.

This book is written by Dr. Richard Scepura, who has authentic experience in burnout, its consequences, and solutions to improve higher functioning at work, and more importantly, higher quality of life. His unique view of the problems we face and the solutions we have at our disposal make it a must-read for this time. It is also a resource that, like many good reads, can be re-read and continue to offer new significance to the reader as their circumstances change. This makes it an excellent addition to any library and a good gift idea for students entering the workplace, schools, or new professions in our changing world.

Dr. Meg Larson, DNP, FNP-C
Primary Care Provider
Veterans Health Associate Professor, Edinboro University

Introduction

There is a body of evidence that explains burnout as a very real global phenomenon experienced by many people in different fields in the workforce. The numbers of those experiencing burnout are increasing despite the knowledge. "Like a frog jumping into a boiling pot of water," all at once, you may feel the effects of burnout because it may not have been evident to you along the way. But it doesn't just happen all at once. It is similar to a slow-moving python that grips its prey, and with an insidious, gradual hold, it squeezes the living daylights out of you.

The emotional, spiritual, physical, psychological, and educational dimensions of a person are impacted greatly when they experience burnout. Each dimension needs special attention to achieve the self-care that is siphoned from you when burnout occurs, often leaving you feeling powerless. In this delightful and impactful book series I created for you, *The Healing Burnout Guide,* I am inviting you, dear reader, to self-reflect. While burnout is often regarded as happening in the workplace, it may occur in your home as well.

Are you feeling stressed or fatigued from the pandemic? Are you feeling the weight of work overload and the pressure of documentation demand? Are you thinking technology has impacted how you live and work and are unhappy with the many changes? Are you becoming frustrated easily? Do you feel as if your personal and work mission are in conflict? Are you experiencing an ethical dilemma or any moral distress? Has it reached a tipping point where you feel like your compassion and service to others seems insincere, and you just go through the motions of performing tasks at your job? Have you become cynical or depersonalized in your approach with people? If so, then I think this book series will really help you.

In my role as a nurse leader, I have witnessed many employees suffering from the effects of burnout. The benefits of performing self-reflection on the variety of topics included will help you expand your emotional quotient (EQ). You will learn how to set limits and put burnout prevention front and center in your mind. As we meander together, exploring and absorbing perspectives, responding to self-reflection questioning, inspired by artistry, you will truly begin to heal on your workbook journey. Give yourself the time to journal daily. **Do not wait!** I promise the benefits of this journaling book will help you immensely to stave off burnout by learning to improve your self-care strategies. My best wishes as you proceed to make self-care your number one priority.

SEASON TWO

Competent

APRIL 1
Day 91

Open Communication

In order to lead an organization that is successful, we must create environments that begin with trust and open communication. Helping employees understand that their work is important and engaging them with open communication sets the tone. Ensuring that your workers realize the bigger picture and how they fit into the puzzle enables them to understand the company's specific goals. Aligning everyone with effective communication ensures staff are operating from comparable perspectives. Keeping the organization moving forward in similar directions will allow the company to achieve desired outcomes. While effective communication may seem relatively easy, it takes a concerted effort.[99]

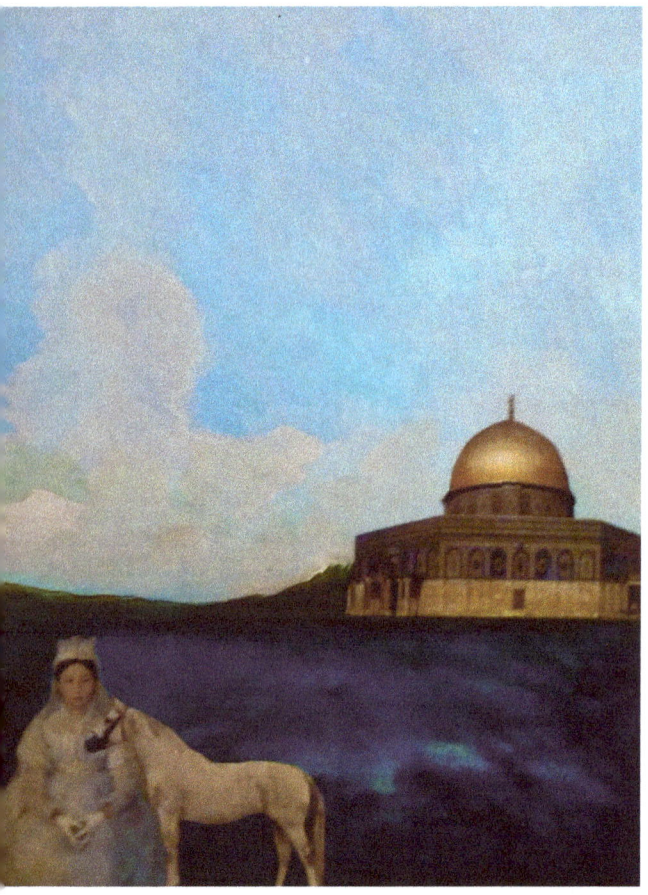

Courtesy of Nancy Nixon Ensign

Today I will consider the communication style at work. Is it open, honest, and free-flowing? Or, is it stifled, guarded, and deliberately suppressed? When communication isn't genuine or respectful, one may feel oppressed. Is this type of environment effective? When feeling burdened all the time about communication at work, it can cause daily cumulative stress and lead to burnout. Journal about communication expectations in the workplace that help keep everyone aligned with the mission.

APRIL 2

Day 92

Celebrating Success

The holidays aren't the only time to have work celebrations. Regular festivities ought to happen all year through. Recognize when your peers go above and beyond, take note, and reward others' successes. Even a small gesture, such as a thank you note, acknowledges hard work with celebration and appreciation which goes a long way.[100]

Today I will consider that we need to celebrate more often, especially within the workplace. When one of my teammates or I have a success, it's important to take the time and acknowledge the milestones – this shows that individuals matter. When we hurriedly keep to the grindstone and don't take a moment to celebrate, the workplace becomes impersonal. Journal about a celebration you have in mind. Is there someone that you want to recognize for their success? Maybe it's your success that you would like others to share in celebrating.

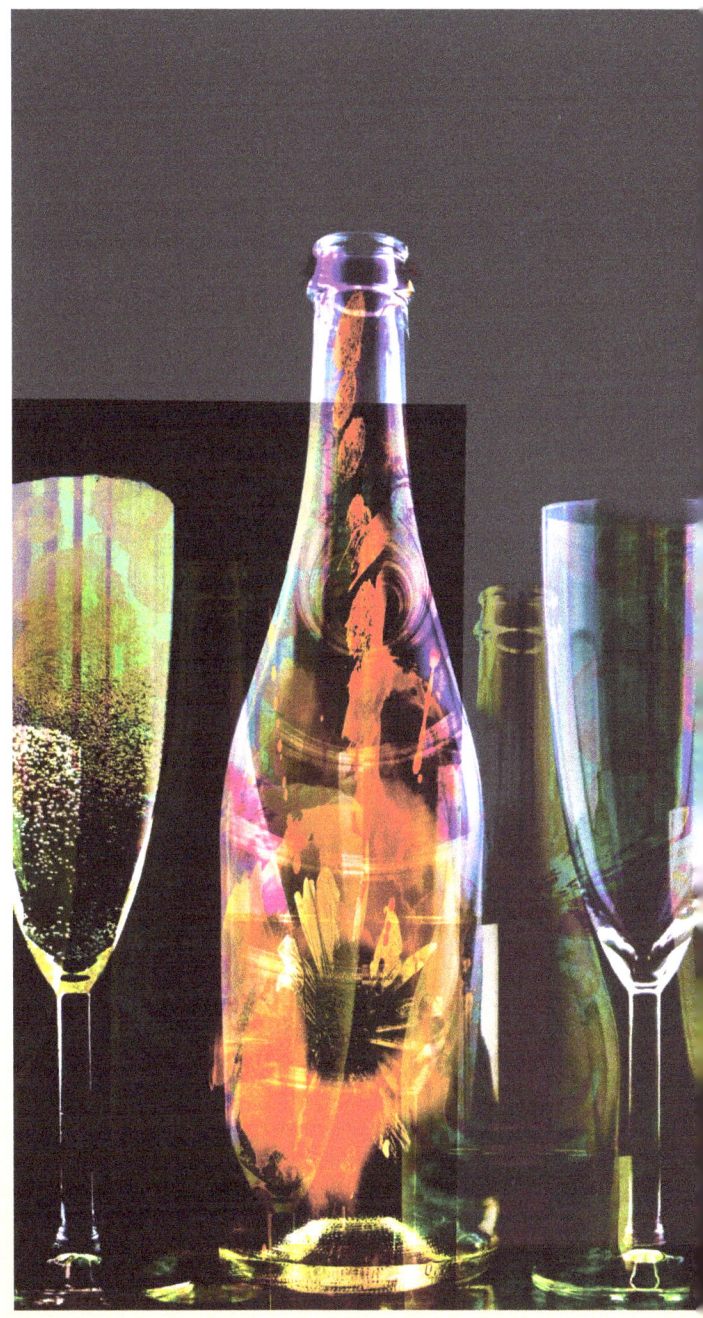

Courtesy of Carrie Shank

APRIL 3

Day 93

Innovation

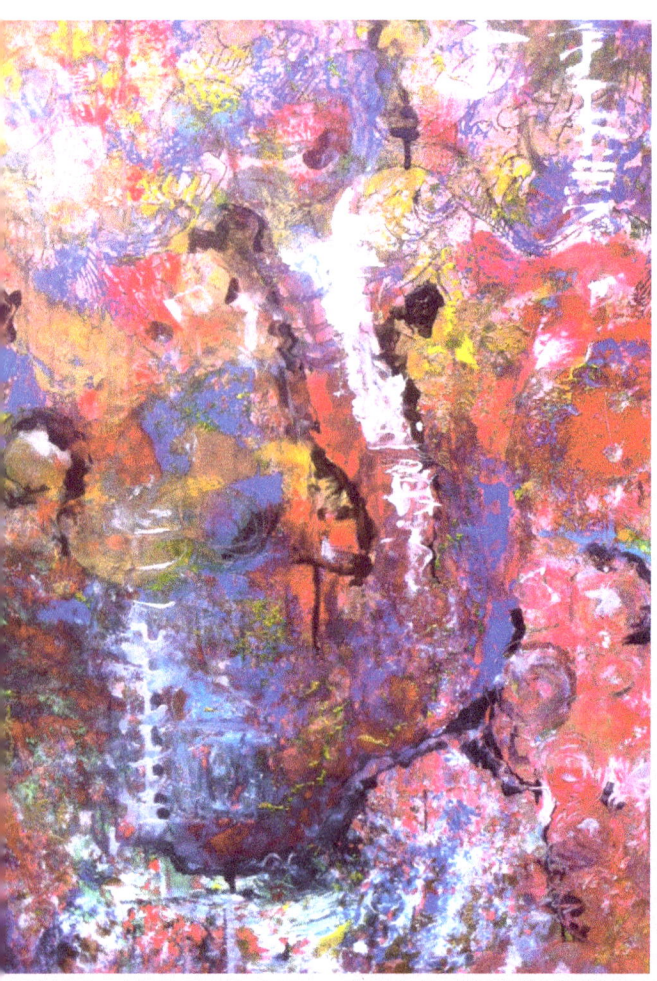
Courtesy of Peter Sterling Turner

With many jobs, there is the risk of developing burnout. When you have a job with high stress and a demanding cognitive load, you are at an increased risk. Scientists, entrepreneurs, and healthcare workers are a few examples of people who experience a high level of mental stress. When employees develop burnout, they may also have increased numbers of substance abuse, depression, divorce, heart disease, or suicide. Workplace errors may become a challenge for those that are burned out. Many depend on "habit memory," where they act reflexively, instead of using "cognitive flexible memory," which carefully examines and weighs factors before acting. Burnout can be a huge problem for innovation economies, including biomedical research and healthcare. Maintaining wellness and being innovative (to prevent excessive stress leading to burnout) is the desired outcome, and creative solutions are necessary.[101]

Today think about stress and how it impacts creativity. If you are stressed most of the time, does this provide a space to be innovative? There is such a thing as positive stress when facing a new challenge. However, not tending to self-care activities only increases negative stress, lack of innovation, and may lead to feelings of burnout. Journal about your creative innovation. How can you carve out a space or time to rejuvenate and get the creative juices flowing? Thinking about a creative space or place for innovation in the home can be as simple as having a comfortable reading corner.

APRIL 4

Day 94

Adaptability

Think of adaptability as having the aptitude for change instead of accepting the status quo and remaining stuck in the past. Our past is what used to be. It contains our memories for reflection and lessons to build on. It cannot be a place for us to reside. Evolving is the result of change. Change guides us to our future. It is a flowing, functional directive in life that nature masterfully understands.[102]

Today I will consider how adaptable I am. Change is the only thing we can count on. If you resist change, you may be passed by and rendered obsolete. Keeping up with change is advised. Journal about your adaptability and your natural reaction toward change. Do you embrace or resist it? Sometimes you don't need to change. If it's not broken, why fix it?

Courtesy of Robert John Holland

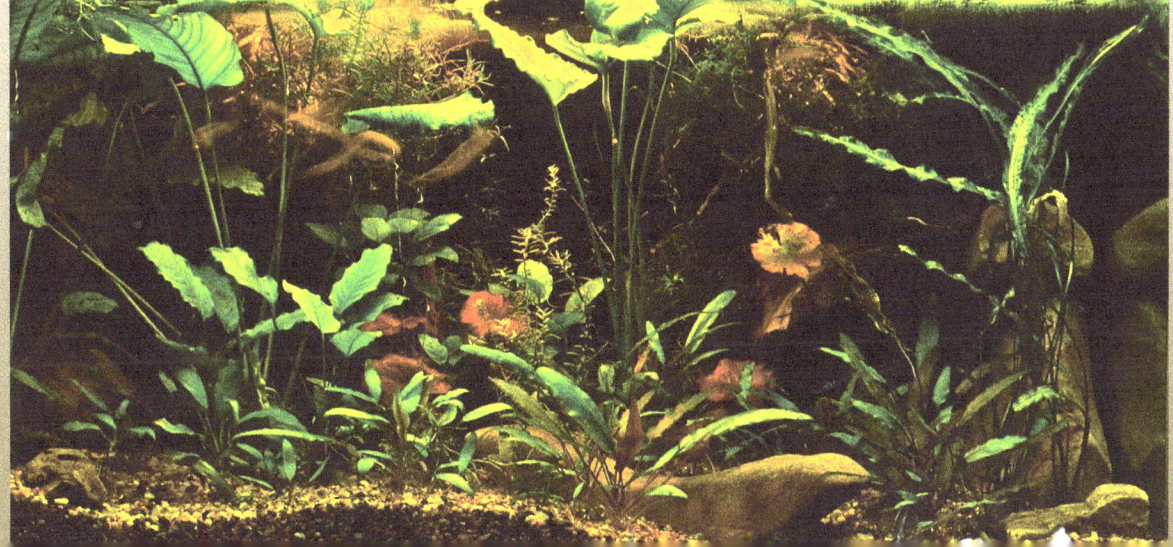

APRIL 5

Day 95

Creating Value

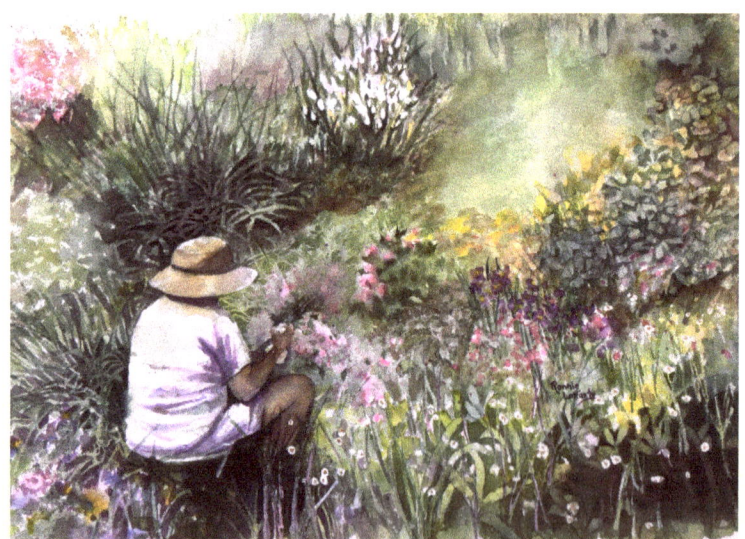

Courtesy of Ronnie Lafferty

Creating true value is about understanding what your client recognizes as valuable. You must also learn to identify how the client views your product versus what competitors have to offer. Do you know what is important to the customer's buying decisions? Do your customers only look at price, or are perceived benefits more important to them? Are you making sure you deliver what the client believes to be important? Are you able to offer and create more value than your competitor?[103]

Today I will consider the value that I contribute to the workplace. Maybe I am not recognized as much as I should be. I will recognize myself. Do you give your clients what they are seeking? Do you deliver value at work? In your journal, reflect on how competition may cause stress despite an organizational need to create and produce valuable outcomes.

APRIL 6

Day 96

Mentorship

Courtesy of Toni Kelly

It has been found that mentorship can mitigate stress and have overall positive effects. In one study, an increased sense of personal accomplishment was achieved after implementing a mentorship program. Both mentors and mentees viewed the program as constructive, and multiple benefits were noted as a result.[104]

Today I will consider finding a mentor if I don't have one. Mentors can be helpful in the short term for specific needs or knowledge gaps you might have, or they can be long term supportive coaches. Knowing what you want help with beforehand is beneficial for your mentorship relationship so that both parties may focus on tailored needs. Finding and working with a mentor may help relieve some stress and lower your chances of burnout. Journal about your mentor relationship or your plan to find mentorship.

Day 97

APRIL 7

Sponsorship

Engaging with a sponsor may help advance your career and can be very useful.[105] Underrepresented minorities, including women, may have opportunities to be mentored; however, sponsoring continues to be low. Sponsorship can help some minorities find employment, raises, promotions, or financial support. Are there ways to find or offer sponsorship of women and marginalized minorities, helping them access greater opportunities to succeed? Diversity can be beneficial for minorities, for the organization, and those working within it. A company that promotes inclusion and diversity at work has the advantage of obtaining many viewpoints, increasing adaptability, and accessing new ideas and perspectives.[106]

Today I will consider whether I need to seek out sponsorship. If I am a minority member, perhaps it is a good idea, as there are many biases. Breaking the glass ceiling may seem nearly impossible and stressful at times, which can lead to additional burnout. Journal about any experiences with employment barriers and how a sponsor might help.

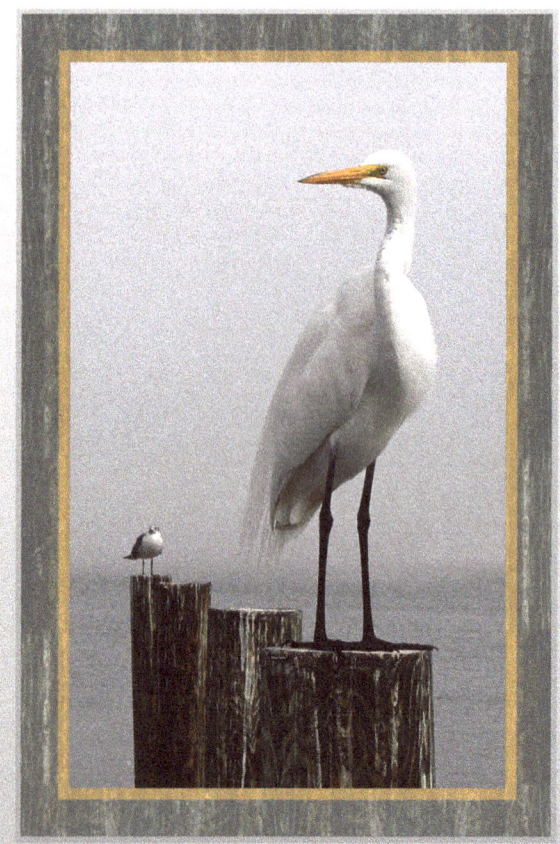

Courtesy of Rebecca Samler

APRIL 8

Day 98

Emotional Intelligence

Understanding emotions and how they guide behaviors is helpful. Recognizing certain emotions in yourself and others and using that knowledge to motivate others is equivalent to your emotional intelligence. When emotional intelligence is lacking with the senior leadership, it is disruptive to the entire work setting. There is a trickle down effect when leaders treat their teams poorly, leading to ineffective states in the work culture. If there are toxic situations happening at work, this may result in high turnover and low engagement. When emotional intelligence is low, morale can be a challenge, causing those who are currently motivated and comfortable to become dissatisfied. When leaders have multiple negative interactions, it may be a sign that they need some work on emotion management.[107]

Today I will consider my interactions with others at work. Answer these questions in your journal. Do you frequently get into 'tetes de tetes' with people? Or are you more tolerant and observant of others? When you are self-aware and socially conscious of what is happening around you, it can be a very positive way to maintain your position or achieve upward movement in your career. Are you conscientious? Are you open to change? How is the emotional intelligence among the senior team where you work?

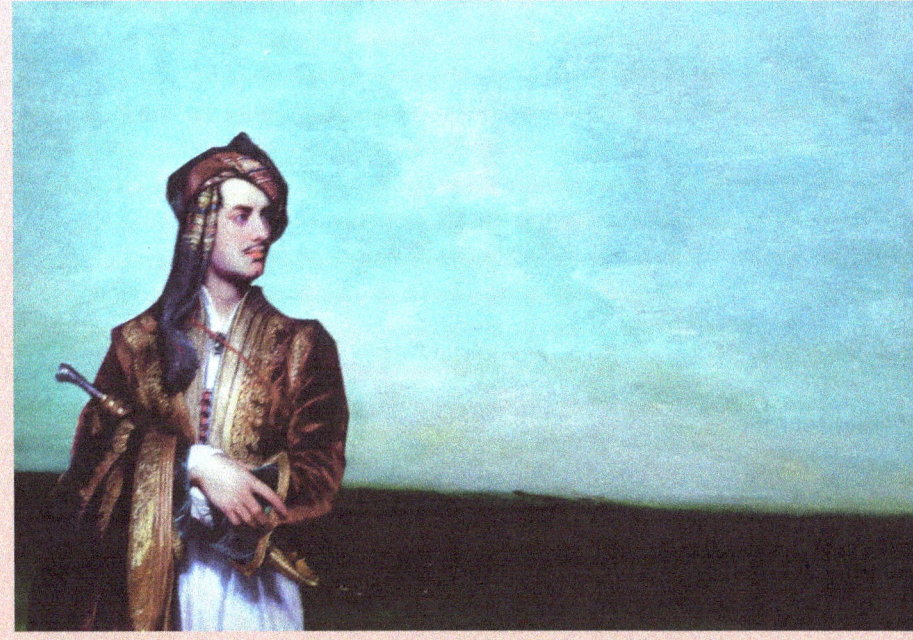

Courtesy of Nancy Nixon Ensign

APRIL 9

Day 99

Burnout and Suicide

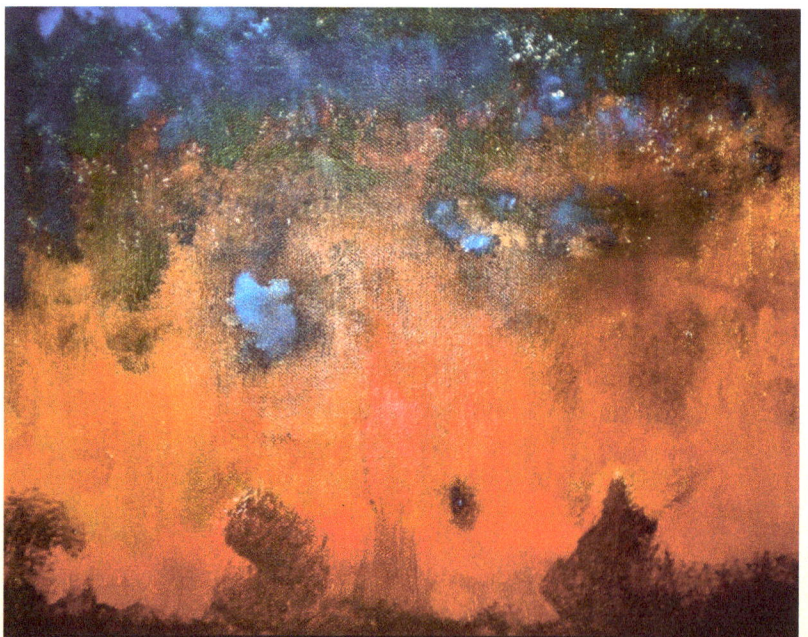

Courtesy of Peter Sterling Turner

The rate of burnout is increasing among many industries. Burnout is on the rise with health providers, social workers, police officers, firefighters, financial analysts, lawyers, and teachers. Dentists have suicide rates that are rising in a similar fashion. The association between burnout and suicide is most apparent. Burnout can elicit feelings of hopelessness and helplessness, which are two major factors involved with depression. It should be clear that depression may lead to suicide and is a significant red flag for those who are suffering burnout versus those who are overly stressed.[108]

Today I will consider whether I or someone I know needs to call the National Suicide Lifeline at 1-800-273-8255 and talk with a counselor about depression, anxiety, or any thoughts of suicide. No job is worth the cumulative and severe effects of burnout. You are worth so much more and can get help. Are your depression and anxiety becoming severe? Journal about steps you can take to overcome these feelings and whether you need to seek help.

APRIL 10

Day 100

Feeling Irritable

It is important to understand that feeling irritable may be a lot more than just an off or upsetting day. There may be underlying issues involved with mental health when habitual irritability is present. Anxiety and depression are two common factors that link to burnout. When irritability is stemming from burnout, a person may feel unimportant, ineffective, or useless. One experiences a sense that they are unable to do things as effectively as before. Early on, irritability related to burnout begins to harm professional and personal interactions. As burnout progresses, it devastates careers and relationships.[109]

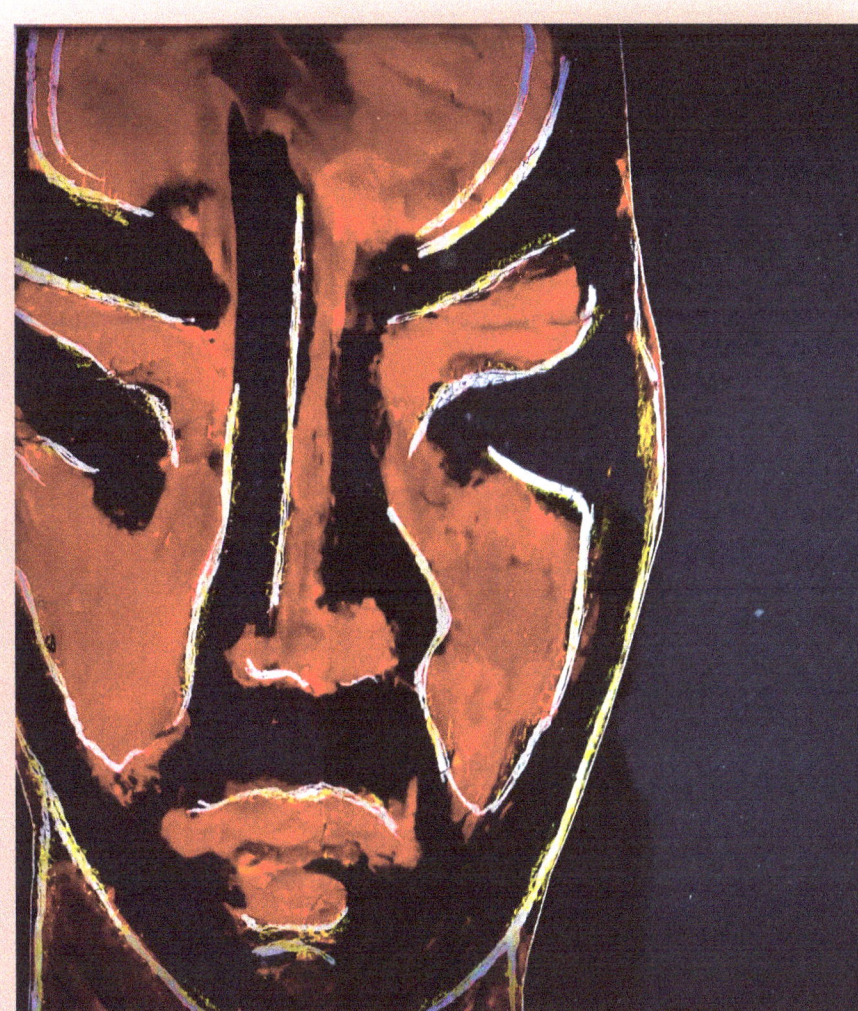

Courtesy of Nancy Nixon Ensign

Today, I will consider my level of irritability. How often do you become irritable? Are you irritable for the sake of being irritable, or is it organic/biochemical? How does it affect coworkers in the work environment? Journal about what it would be like to share your thoughts about your irritability with a supportive person. What would help to reduce your tension? Are there things at home you can try like mindfulness, deep breathing, yoga, boxing, aromatherapy, reading a book, or nature walks?

APRIL 11

Day 101

Regaining Peace

Peace is often thought of as a destination, like imagining eventually achieving happiness and success. It is viewed as something we need to find or chase after, as opposed to something that can be experienced without drastically changing your life. Many desire working less while relaxing more, or revamping relationships and circumstances to become a more peaceful person. However, it is important to realize that although peace may always be available, like any preferable mindset, it requires actual effort, including the conscious decision to choose stillness.[110]

Today I will take a moment and be still. Find the time, regardless of the calamity happening at home or at work, to regain your peace. Being deliberate when you do this contributes to your happiness. What you consciously choose makes you successful. When you do not have moments of calm, your stress grows, which in time can lead to burnout. Journal about regaining your sense of peace. What things bring you peace and help you create calm?

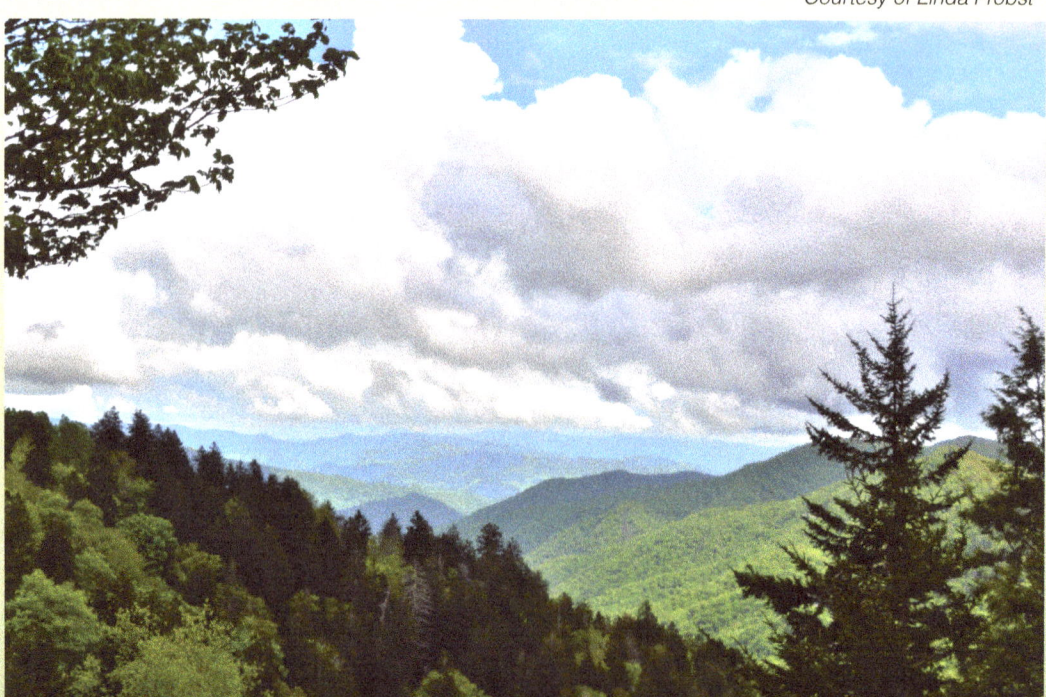

Courtesy of Linda Probst

APRIL 12

Day 102

Friendship at Work

The effect of social interaction on positive wellbeing is linked directly. Common concerns regarding personal relationships in the workplace make understanding your friendships in a professional environment quite confusing. Companies want to promote employees to be productive and successful. They also try to prevent inappropriate behavior from happening. Common examples of what can occur from inappropriate behaviors and relationships within the workplace include favoritism, harassment, authoritative abuse, or conflicts of interest. In these times, where workers are driven by both career and their own wellness, finding a healthy balance with relationships in the workplace is of the utmost importance.[111]

Today I will think about my friendships at work. Are you overly friendly with your coworkers, or do you have a healthy balance? Getting support from friends at work can be a good thing. However, unchecked relationships can be overly enmeshed or create a conflict of interest. Keeping a healthy distance and professional boundaries can help prevent awkward and unnecessary stressors at work. This is beneficial in creating a healthy network of friends. Journal about who you are friendly with at work and whether it is a healthy, balanced relationship.

Courtesy of Toni Kelly

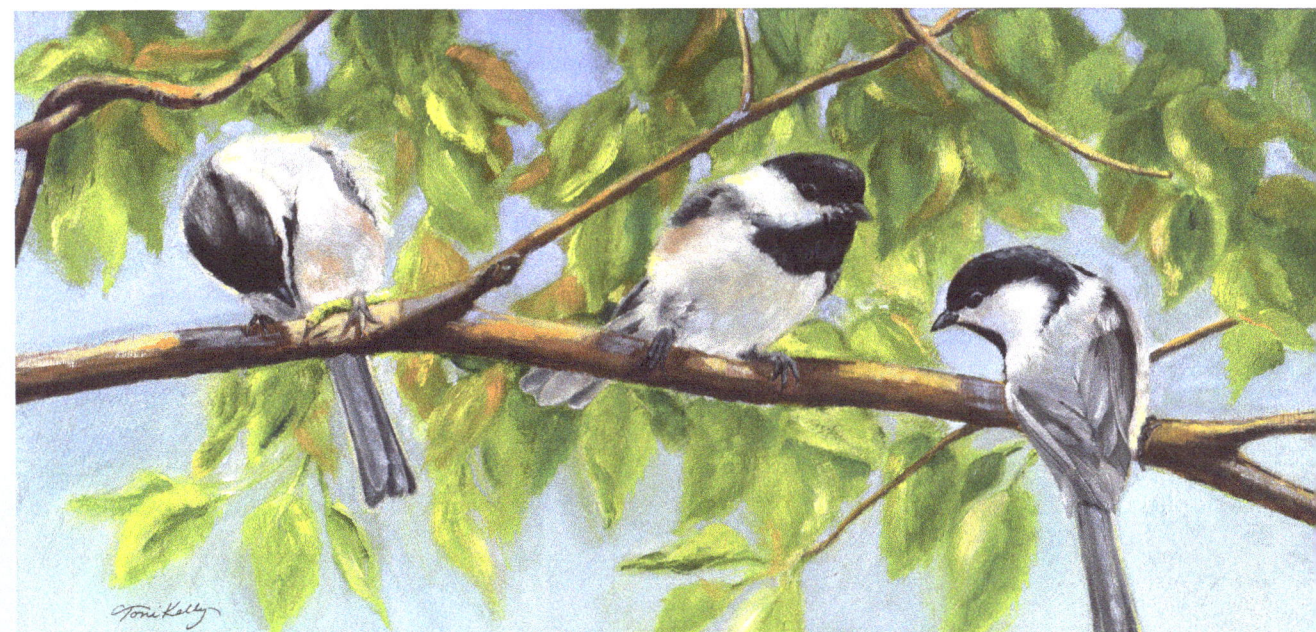

APRIL 13

Day 103

Humanity

Today's healthcare system is unable to be sustained without a healthy workforce or restored humanity. The clinician's wellness is imperative so that they can perform their professional role. The companies where clinicians work must be responsible for protecting and preserving their wellness by creating systems that encourage it. Ethically, it is not justified to ignore the very real outcomes of systems in crisis. Being able to recognize burnout among nurses and doctors is urgent. Clinicians are responsible for caring for those who are most vulnerable. Therefore, investing in them is a must to continue bringing their talent and gifts to those who need it most.[112]

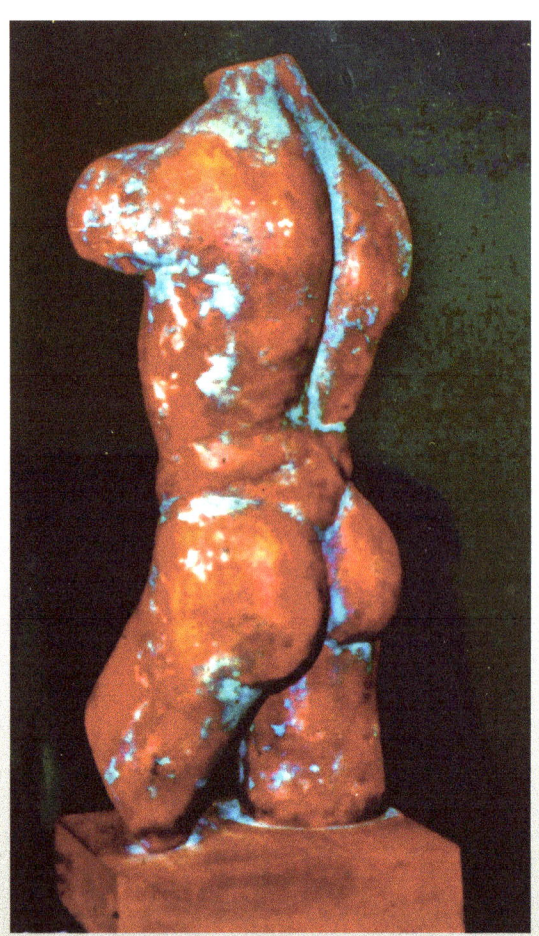

Courtesy of Nancy Nixon Ensign

Today I will take notice of what things my organization is doing to address burnout in the workplace. Those are the things that restore faith in humanity. Write down as many things as you can in your journal. If you cannot identify anything that your organization is doing to ameliorate burnout, perhaps ask your manager, director, or human resource representative, and see what they say. While some organizations may have activities and plans in place to combat burnout, others may not.

APRIL 14

Day 104

Soft Skills

Possessing soft skills means you are more likely to adapt and learn easily over someone without them. Soft skills can be a major factor in building relationships, creating opportunities, or developing advancement through your creativity. No matter how hard you try at work, it is still those soft skills that make the difference for you. Without them, the chance of succeeding in your career is very minimal.[113]

Today I will consider my overall demeanor. Are you gentle, friendly, and easily able to forge relationships? Are you included in projects, and do people seek out your opinion? Be realistic about your soft skills and learn about the subject, especially if you are not advancing and dissatisfied because no promotion is in sight. How does stress impact your soft skills? How does burnout impact your soft skills? Journal about that now.

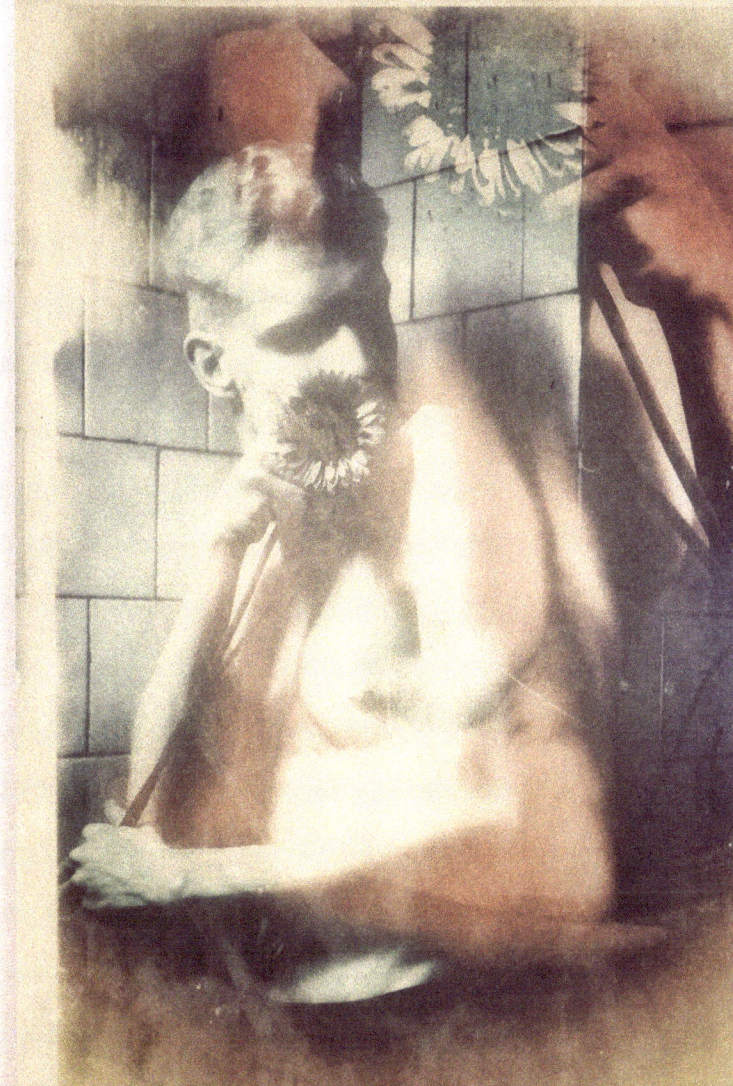

Courtesy of Carrie Shank

APRIL 15

Day 105

Finding Joy Through Work

Joy is diminished within the healthcare workforce because of the same concerns that increase burnout. Leaders in healthcare must understand which factors are diminishing workplace joy while also nurturing their employees and act on the issues that create burnout. The most engaged and productive staff feel both psychologically and physically safe. The purpose and meaning of their work are very important to them, as well as having choices and control over their time. They encounter camaraderie when work is viewed as being equitable and fair.[114]

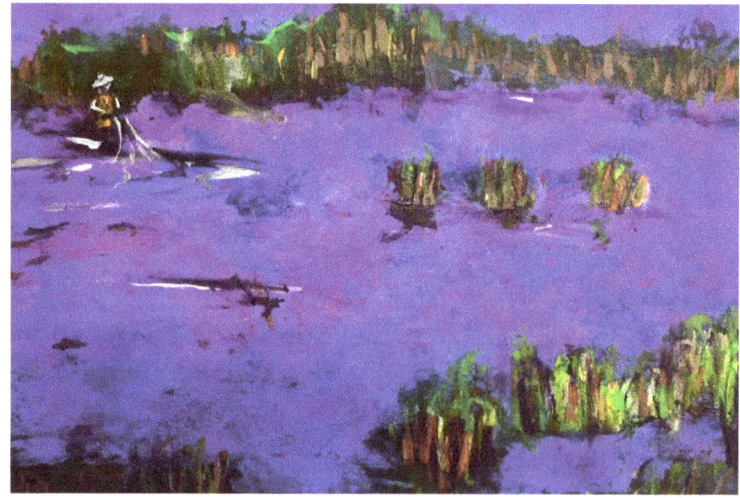

Courtesy of Peter Sterling Turner

Today I will think about whether my work brings me joy. Being realistic and understanding the reasons why you stay in your job is helpful to know. For instance, if you stay because your job brings you joy, that is great. What are the other reasons for staying if you are not experiencing happiness at work? List some reasons in your journal and think about plans you can make to find joy again. Carefully consider your options.

APRIL 16

Day 106

Exclusion from Decision Making

Have you ever felt isolated on the job? Whether you were omitted from a meeting or your ideas fell on deaf ears, you must find a way to raise concerns, despite not being invited to voice your opinion. If speaking your thoughts receives pushback or resistance, and you are given negative responses from a colleague or supervisor, you might want to reassess how the company values you. Don't let your talents be suppressed or undermined. If these things are unsuccessful, you may realize your workplace is not the right fit.[115]

Today I will consider when the last time was that I attended a meeting or conference. What was your manner like? Were you quiet and non-participative? Or were you engaging and bringing forth ideas? Journal about whether you are included or excluded from the decision-making processes at work. How does this make you think or feel?

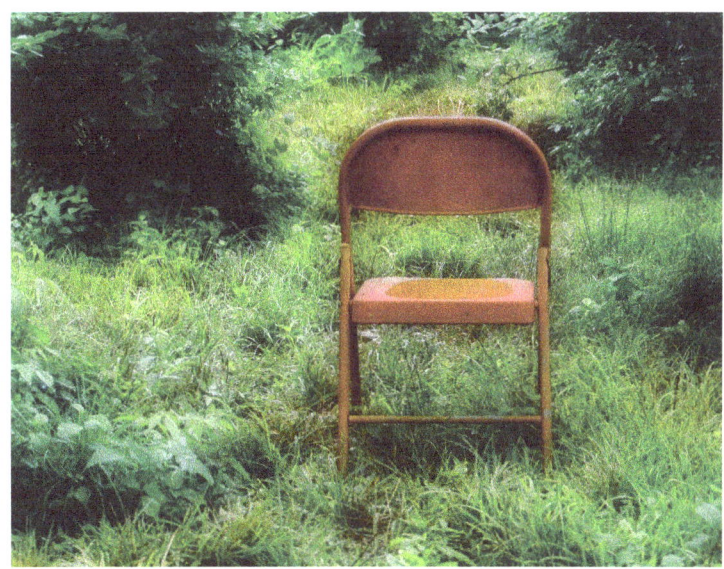

Courtesy of Ann Parker

APRIL 17

Day 107

Violence in the Workplace

OSHA surveys indicate about 2 million American workers each year become victims of violence within the workplace. No one is exempt from workplace violence. There are certain workers who tend to be at increased risk, however. These include those who deal directly with clients or customers, exchanging money, transporting passengers, working by themselves or with others in small groups. They work all hours of the day, around the clock. Their job can bring them to areas where high crime occurs or in community homes and settings. Examples of these workers include those in social services or healthcare, such as home-care nurses, probation officers, or psychiatric evaluators. Also included are gas and water utility employees, cable and phone installers, mail carriers, workers in retail, and cab drivers.[116]

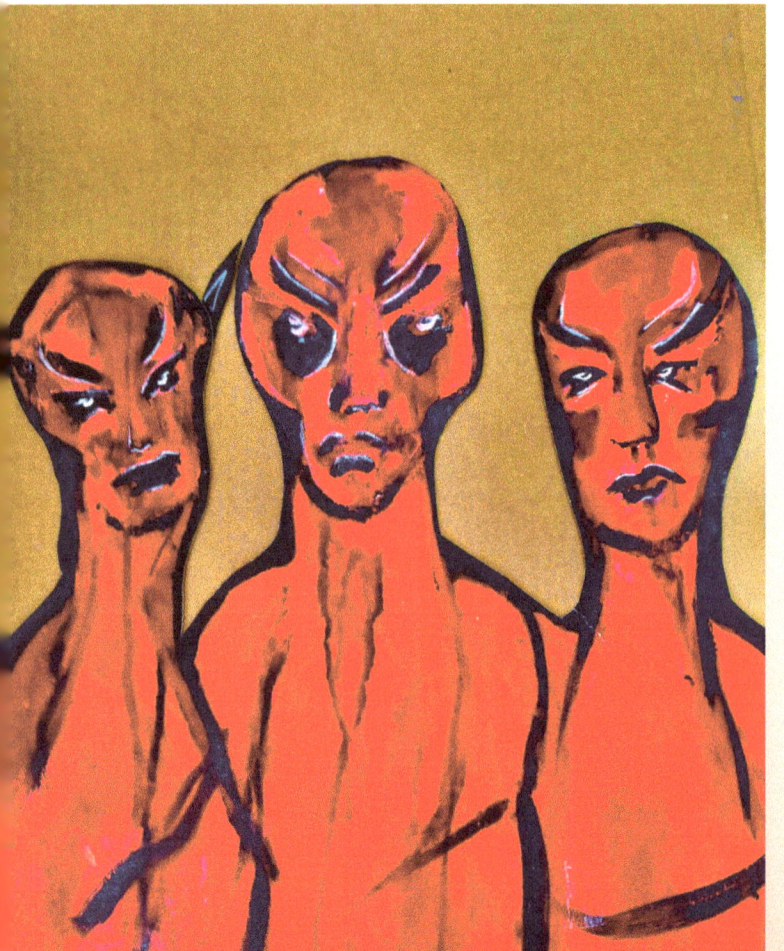

Courtesy of Nancy Nixon Ensign

Today I will consider my risk of exposure to violence in the workplace, which may be unavoidable. Have you witnessed violence in the workplace? If you work in one of these high exposure areas, how does this contribute to your stress and eventual burnout? Does your employer have a zero-tolerance policy for violence? Prompt attention to workplace violence is essential in decreasing occurrences. Write about your thoughts and answers in your journal.

APRIL 18
Day 108

Need for Greater Autonomy

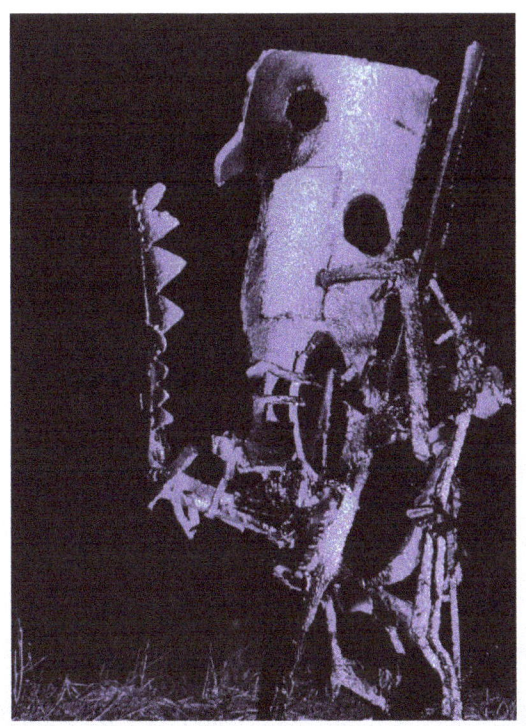

Courtesy of Robert John Holland

Autonomy is about granting workers their freedom of creativity. Allow them to choose where, when, and how they complete their work. Enable employees to display their own thoughts and ideas, develop their personal objectives, and have the confidence to try new approaches. Give workers the encouragement and distance they need to capture new ideas while allowing them to connect with the values that inspire their work. From a creative point of view, autonomy allows everyone to feel empowered.[117]

Today I will consider exactly how much autonomy I have at work. A little? A lot? Do people give you space at work so you can be creative? Or do you follow the same protocol day in and day out because that is what is asked of you? If the latter, what is your plan for coping with monotony? Some people might not mind doing the same thing day in and day out. Do you? Journal about your autonomy and how you can inject some creativity into your daily routine to help avoid burnout from repetition.

APRIL 19

Day 109

Entrepreneurship

It is common for entrepreneurs to face burnout. Entrepreneurs are recognized for their extremely hard work in order to achieve success within their business. The demands that entrepreneurship entails, both real and self-imposed, together with excruciating schedules and deadlines they face, often lead to long-term stress and burnout.[118]

Today I will consider entrepreneurship. Is there an opportunity for you to create your own business? If so, starting a business venture will require long hours until you are established. Journal about the following questions. How will you combat the stress? What self-care activities do you enjoy and are prepared to do? Perhaps having a joint entrepreneur and self-care plan is in order.

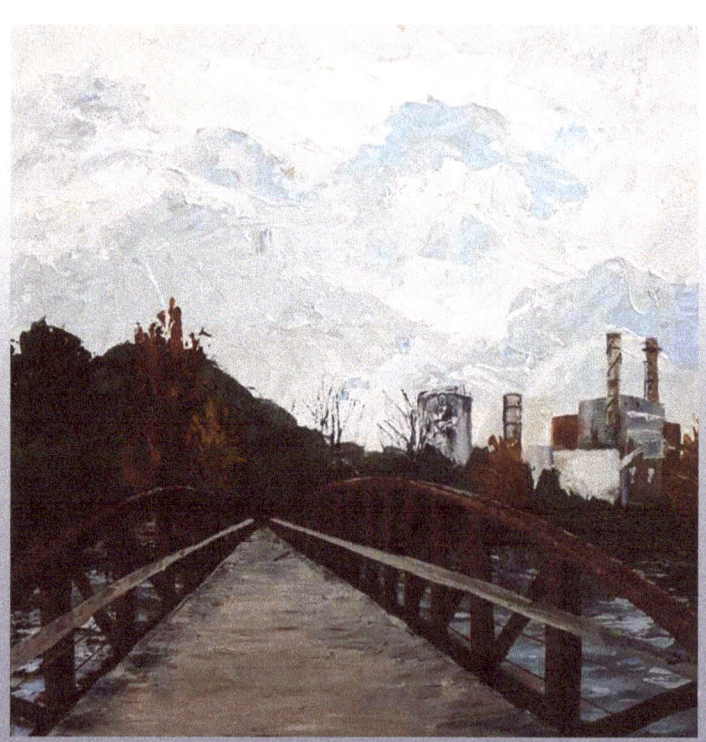
Courtesy of Susan Gutierrez

Day 110 — **APRIL 20**

Shining at Work

The happiest and most successful people truly thrive on what they do in their careers. Investing in what matters and focusing energy towards being the best is "shining at work." How can you become someone who does more than just show up to work and go through the motions? By being someone who exceeds expectations and excels at what you are doing. Shining in your work environment can be difficult to achieve, especially when working within a large group or for a business where excellency is status quo and an expectation.[119]

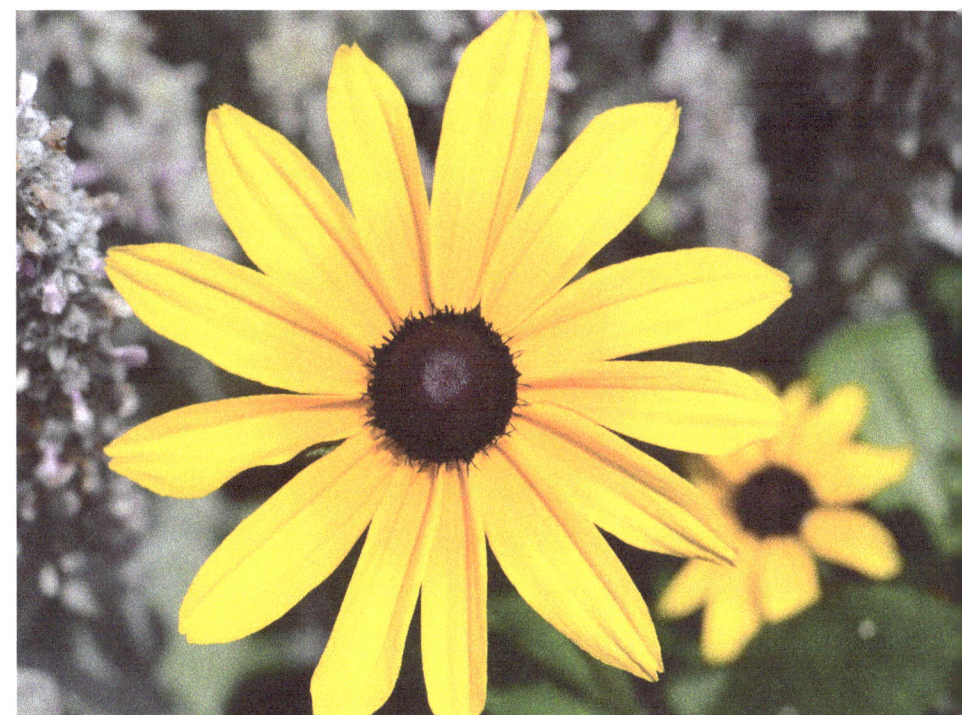

Courtesy of Jill Santi

Today I will think about how I "shine" at my workplace. Even if others don't notice how I shine, I will notice and reward myself. In today's hurried and overburdened work environments, people don't always take the time to recognize each other. Journal about how you can recognize others that shine and how you would like to be recognized.

APRIL 21

Day 111

Resilience

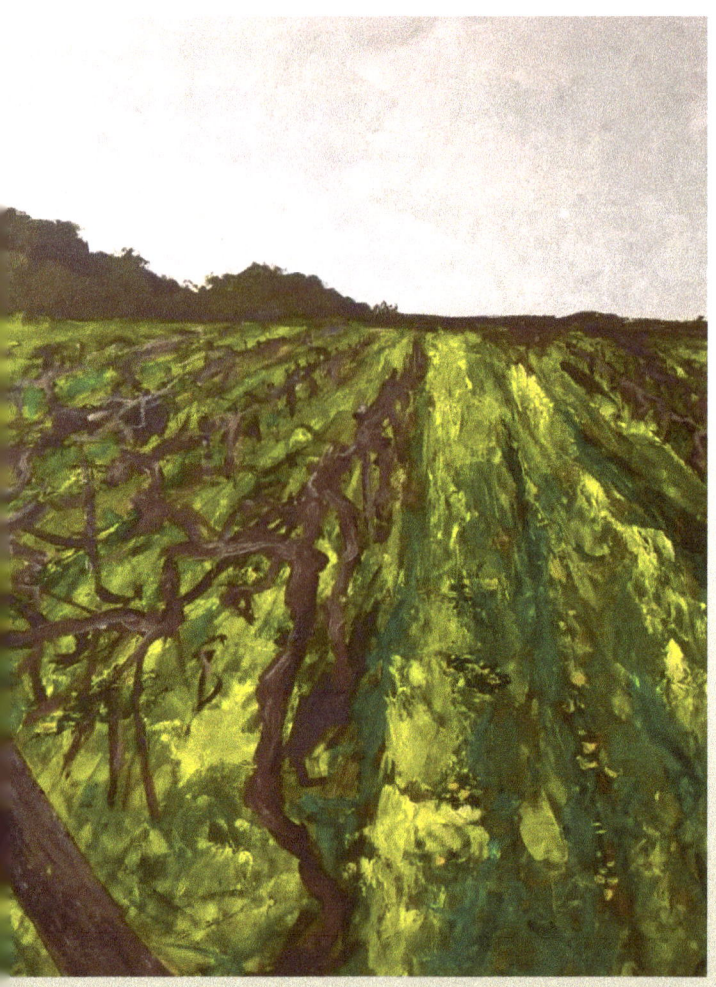

Courtesy of Susan Gutierrez

When burnout concerns increase and begin to gather attention, suggestions for building resilience, minimizing stress, and increasing mindfulness tend to be everywhere. You should not assume that burnout is due to a lack of flexibility. Resilience, the ability to recover from difficult times, is a requirement to become a clinician. "Ironically, the path to heal others can harm those who walk along it." We must redesign resilience training as a form of growth while experiencing stress. It just so happens that some very resilient, kind people have been clearly overworked. Healthcare, with its many challenges and demands, has "score carded" out the caring for human beings.[120]

Today I will consider that I may already be resilient if I practice in healthcare and perhaps other professions. Everything I do as a professional requires resilience. Think about some of the ways the workplace exhausts workers. Do you have ideas for fixing some of the things that create exhaustion? What can be reduced, eliminated, revised, kept the same, or improved? Journal about your resilience and how you can help others build it.

APRIL 22

Day 112

Renewal

Merriam-Webster defines renewal as "the state of being made new, fresh, or strong again." It could be said that leadership and follower renewal is the equivalent of feeling complete. Alternatively, the antonym of renewal is the depleted condition of burnout. This means feeling exhausted instead of energized, cynical instead of engaged, or ineffective instead of productive. Leaders need to demonstrate self-renewal, along with looking for ways to encourage revitalization for others. Renewal often requires more than getting a bit of rest. In today's world, we are required to communicate frequently while managing excess data. Our daily lives also consist of an increase in tasks and more to follow-up on than other previous generations. Rest can help renew our strength and energy; however, it doesn't do much to motivate us. If motivation is lacking, we need to rediscover our mission, life's purpose, and rejuvenation for the work we do.[121]

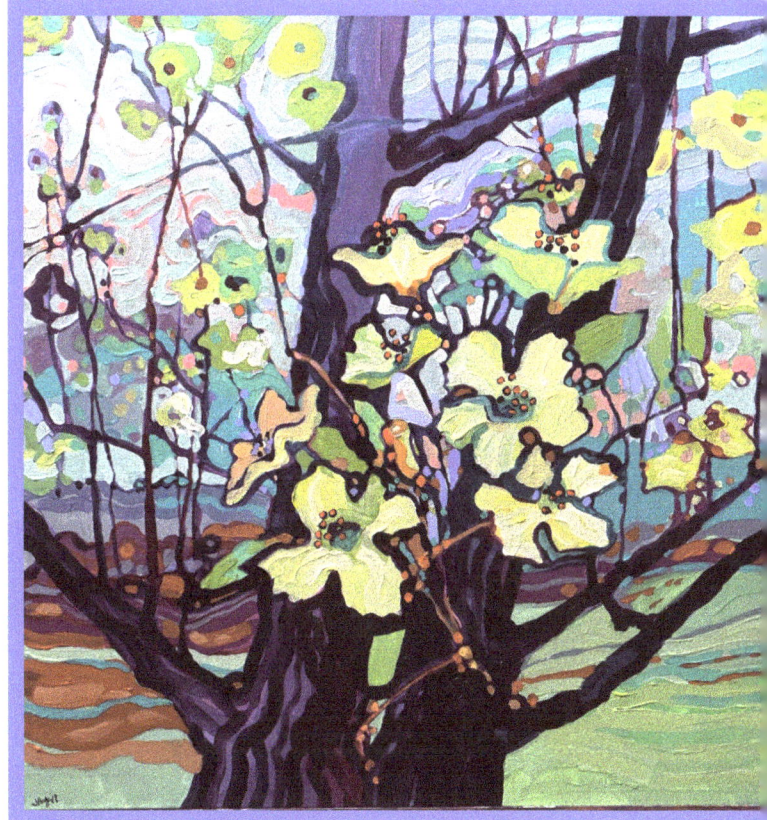

Courtesy of Judy Hodge

Today I will think about renewal. Do you know what your core values and mission are? Take some time to rest and renew, slow down a bit, and regain some strength. How is your motivation? Do you need rejuvenation? What is your energy level? What does renewal mean to you? How can you inspire others to seek it in themselves? Journal about your answers.

APRIL 23

Day 113

Being Gracious

British poet George Herbert stated, "Good words are worth much, and cost little." An example of a good word is the word "grace." Grace is feeling a sense of propriety and fitness. It is also the tendency to be helpful and generous. We do not hear the word "grace" often enough within the workplace, except when an employee has fallen from grace or their behavior is seen as disgraceful. Grace is a key factor that helps bind us with others. Grace is needed when we interact in our relationships with clients, employees, coworkers, friends, or family. Being gracious is the level of civility binding us with strangers. Grace doesn't cost us anything, yet it can buy a lot of goodwill.[122]

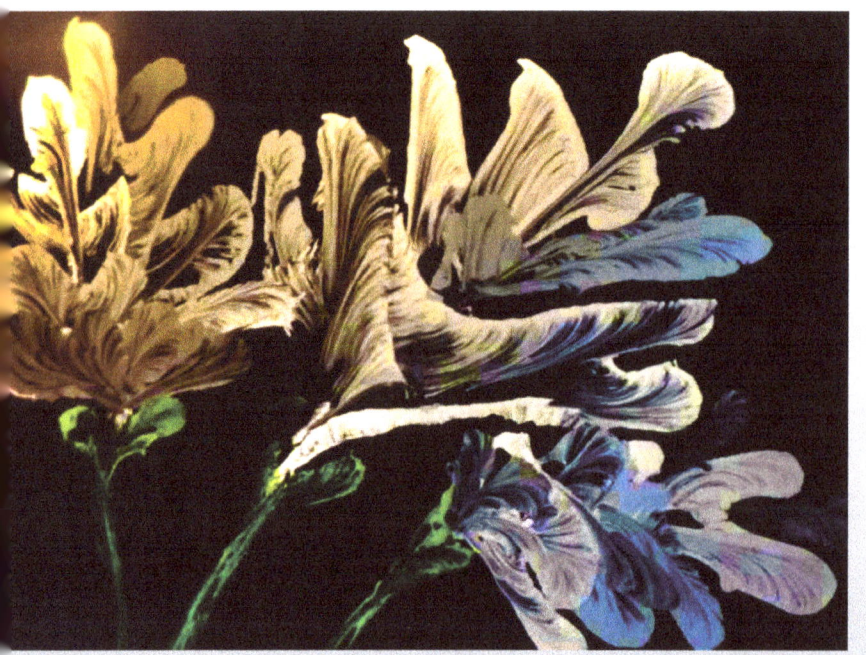

Courtesy of Aryn Grayson

Today and each day, I will be gracious. It doesn't take much and isn't stressful. Remember the English Proverb, "You catch more flies with honey than vinegar." Take notice of when you are gracious or spread goodwill. Journal about whether you choose honey over vinegar in your interactions with people. Are you helpful, generous, and do you role model civility?

APRIL 24
Day 114

Receiving Feedback

If you receive feedback (for example, a performance evaluation of a project you have done recently), you must try and distinguish your skills and traits apart from your entire being. It is much easier to understand small parts of feedback than to assume the criticism is directed towards you personally. It can be difficult not to overanalyze when you receive feedback, yet it is an important skill to evaluate it objectively. Before acting after receiving feedback, try to stop, breathe, and think about what you were told before giving a response.[123]

Today I will remember that receiving feedback doesn't have to be stressful or devastate me. Receiving feedback is accepting another's opinion. Evaluate the feedback. Think about whether you value and incorporate the feedback into better performance. Try to receive feedback without judgment. Journal about how you incorporate feedback into becoming a better version of yourself.

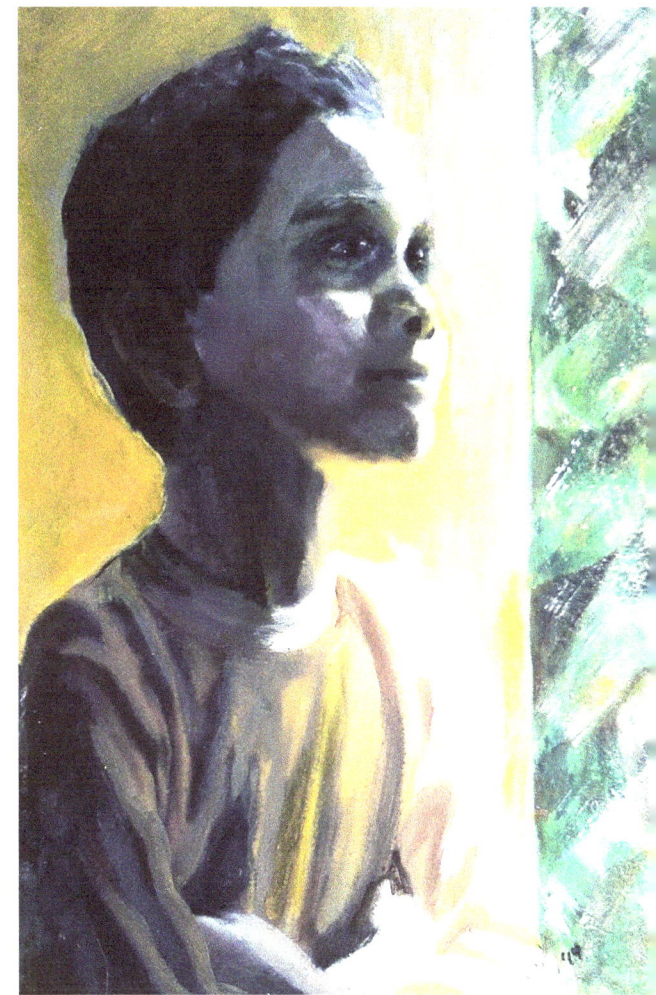

Courtesy of Susan MacKay

APRIL 25

Day 115

Giving Feedback

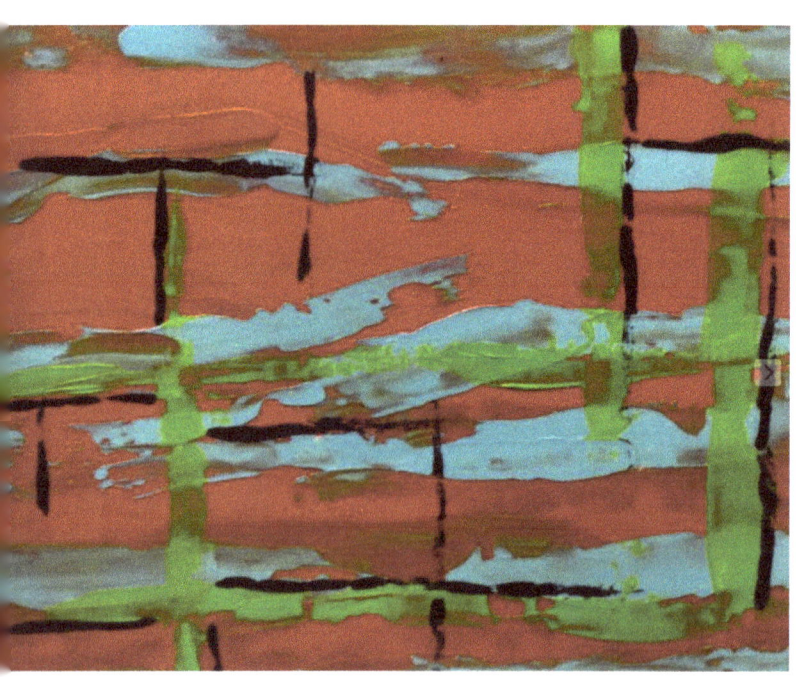

Courtesy of Aryn Grayson

When people receive feedback, they may only apply it 30% of the time. If someone receiving feedback doesn't seem receptive or comfortable with what they are being told, it could ultimately result in the feedback being unproductive. Adding safety and civility to the way you deliver feedback may be helpful. When giving a response to someone, try not to be mean. When your attention is focused on upsetting someone or making them appear foolish in the company of others, your feedback will likely be unproductive.[124]

Today I will consider whether the feedback I give is helpful or harmful. Realize that there is only a 30% chance the person will integrate it into their performance or behavior. Sometimes what we think is meaningful feedback is not objective at all. Rather, it can be harsh and subjective. Journal about how you can plan your feedback and offer helpful advice.

APRIL 26
Day 116

Competitiveness

It is important to focus on improving yourself without being overly competitive or comparing yourself to others. The true comparison that is most important is your self today against what you believe is your ideal self. If visualizing something will help grasp this concept better, think of relationships being horizontal rather than vertical. For example, imagine a stairway where you are climbing up and must push beyond others to get on top. Instead, try replacing that image with a level field in which all people move forward. Some that are moving forward may also be behind you. Those behind you are still making progress, yet everyone is at different stages.[125]

Today I will consider how competitive I am. How might that appear to others? While being competitive is not always a bad thing, it displays behavior around competitiveness that may be concerning, creates stress, and puts people off. Journal about how you perceive your competitiveness. How can you help others while being competitive as well? Offering a hand to those falling behind won't harm you.

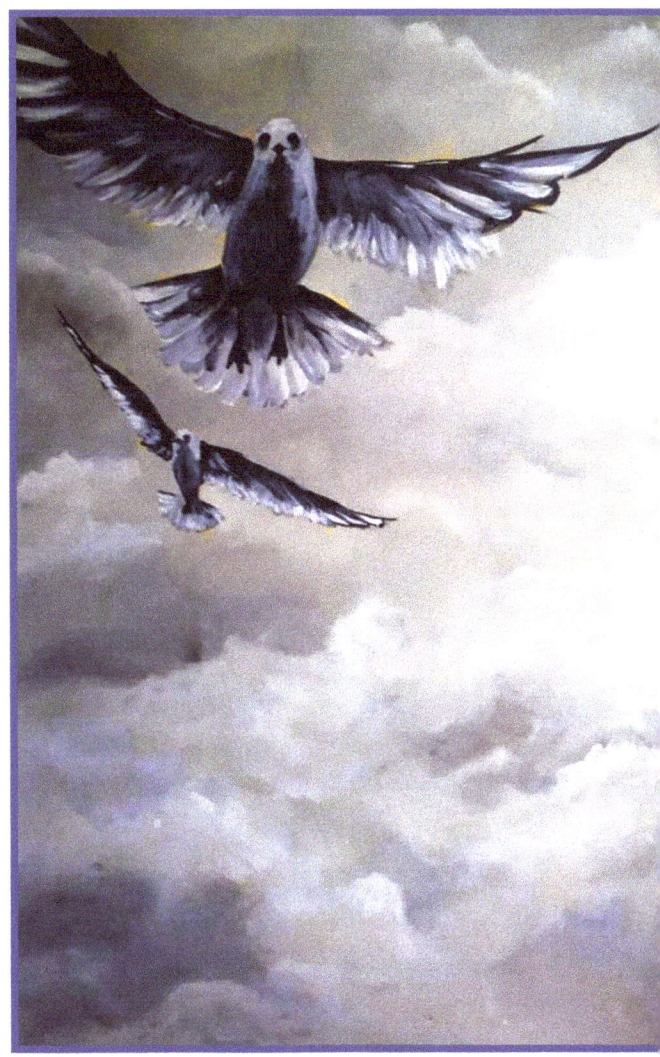

Courtesy of Susan Gutierrez

APRIL 27

Day 117

Support Systems

There are many benefits of using individualized support systems to assist with stress reduction, decrease health problems, and improve your emotional wellness. Taking note of your support systems is a great way to learn exactly where your assistance truly comes from. Who is providing it? Taking stock can also help you understand why you prefer not to request or accept help and reasons why others don't offer it.[126]

Today I will evaluate the support systems that I have in place. Make a list in your journal of those that you can count on. Do you have enough support? If not, where can you get more? Whether it is social, supportive, sport-related, or a hobby, joining a group can be extremely rewarding and offer that piece that is missing in your work-life balance. Journal about a group you can join outside of work or which family and friends you can count on.

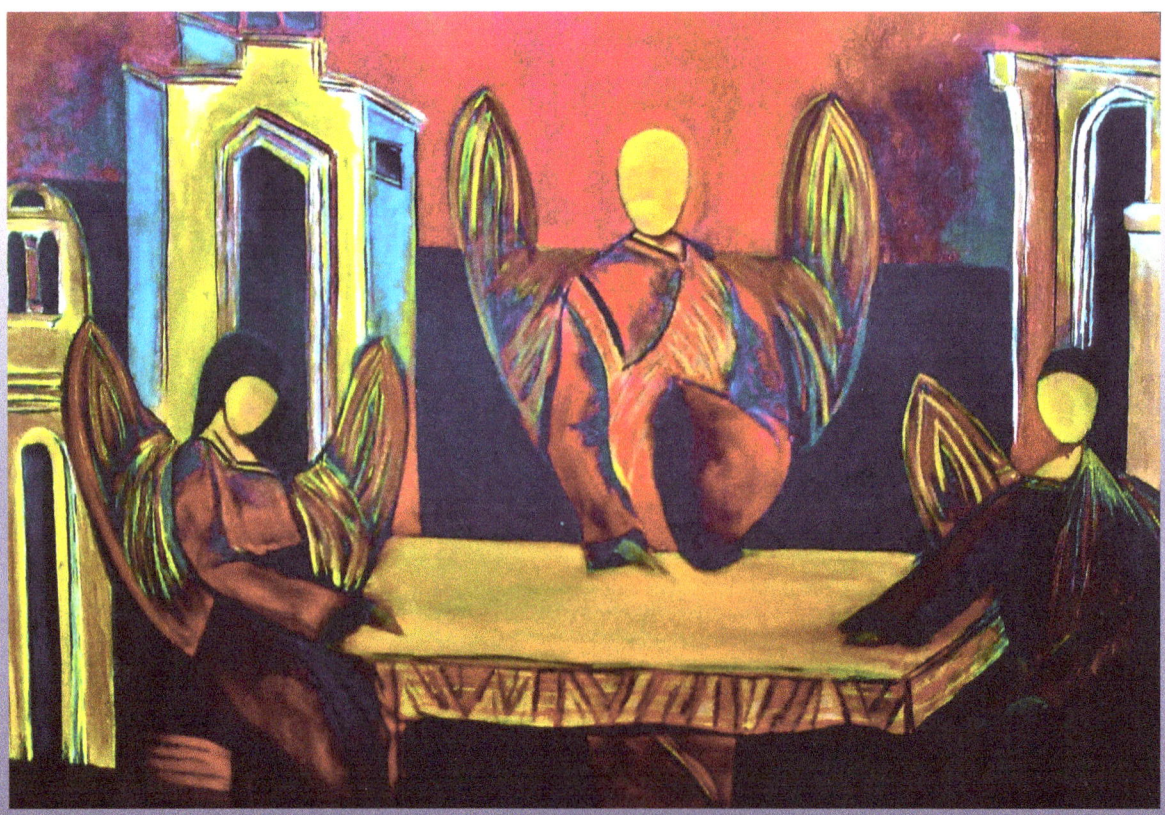

Courtesy of Nancy Nixon Ensign

APRIL 28

Day 118

Dream More

"If your actions create a legacy that inspires others to dream more, learn more, do more, and become more, then you are an excellent leader."[127] — D. Parton

Today I will think about the dreams that I have. Our fast-paced world does not offer us much time to dream. Do you remember your dreams? Do you dream about stressful work-related situations? (This is a sign of burnout). Consider learning more, doing more, and becoming more. However, you are enough as you are today. Journal about how often you dream and the quality of your dreams. Do you dream frequently or infrequently? How can you inspire others to dream more?

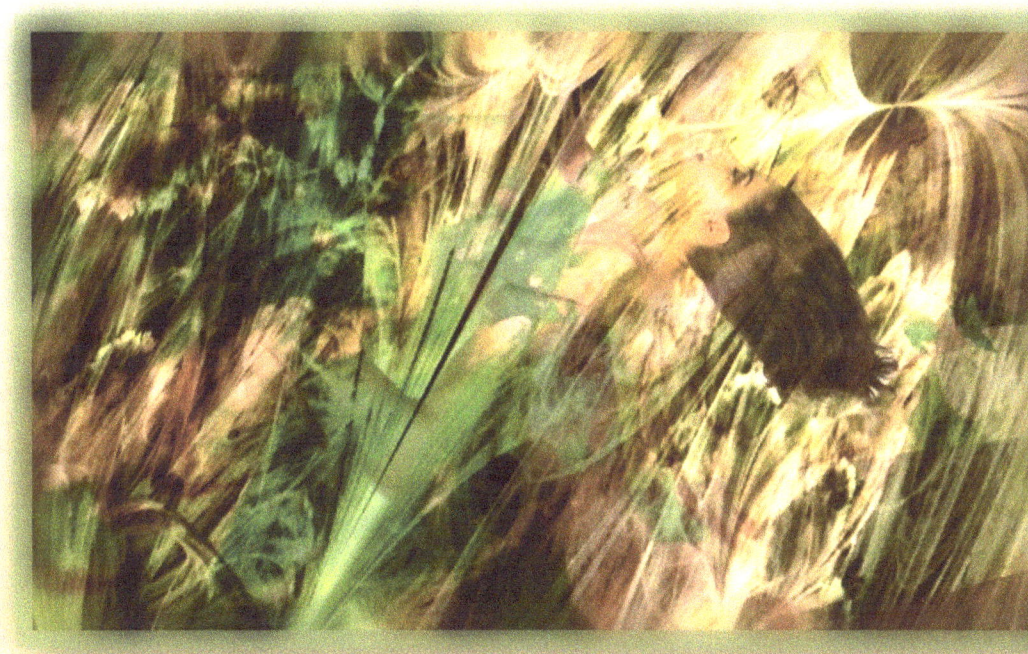

Courtesy of Carrie Shank

APRIL 29
Day 119

Enthusiasm at Work

Employers often want to choose candidates that have the best skills, training, and experiences. Often, they want to hire those that have an upbeat enthusiasm while demonstrating cooperativeness. Candidates with a positive demeanor, and eagerness to get the job done have advantages over those with disinterested attitudes. Employers would rather provide training for those that exhibit enthusiasm at work, even if they are inexperienced, compared with others having the qualifications with a less than stellar attitude. There is some concern by management that a less than positive employee will not be a good teammate and not fit into the culture. The negative employee likely lacks effort in their work, is disrespectful toward coworkers, supervisors, and may even treat customers poorly. However, employees that display enthusiasm at work most likely give excellent service, are effective at solving conflict, and are productive with their team.[128]

Courtesy of Patti Larson

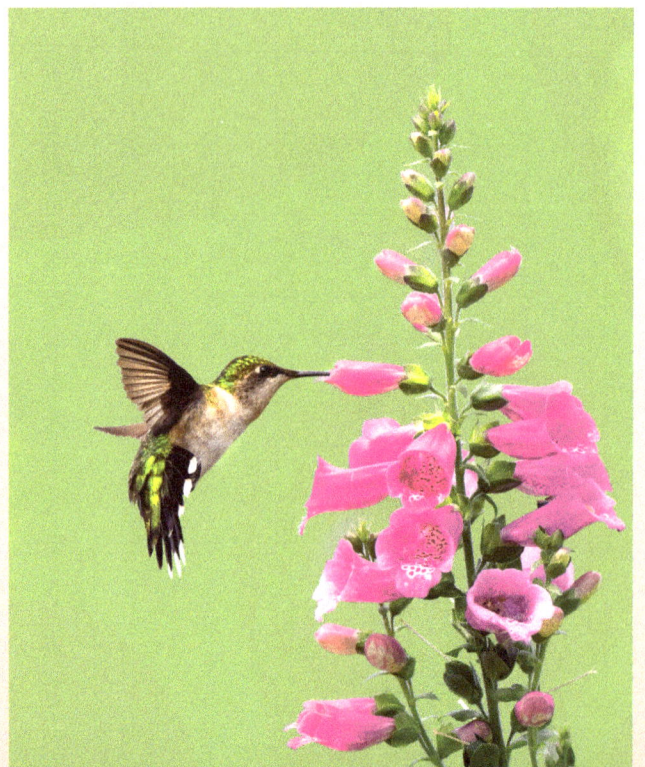

Today I will consider enthusiasm at work. It is not always easy to be enthusiastic while working, especially in high stress areas or life or death circumstances. How do you find the reserves to maintain a positive attitude, eagerness, and good customer service? A keen self-awareness and high emotional quotient are the best tools. Journal about any reserves you may have that bring out an upbeat cooperative persona.

APRIL 30

Day 120

Overcoming Obstacles

Those who overcome obstacles find new perspectives when reflecting on their previous problems. In order to overcome difficulties, try to incorporate creative thinking, which is a skill that makes you successful in other aspects and areas of your life. There is an old cliché that "challenges are simply opportunities." Successful people do not fear failure when they attempt new solutions or look for paths for overcoming obstacles. Remember that failure simply happens in life. Many successful people have dealt with failing publicly.[129]

Today I will consider just how many obstacles I have faced in my life. Journal about the following questions. What is the biggest obstacle of your past? What is the current stressful obstacle you are facing now? What is the biggest obstacle coming downstream? Seeing the obstacles in your path allows you to navigate them. Failing to plan is planning to fail. However, you can choose to turn your failures into successes.

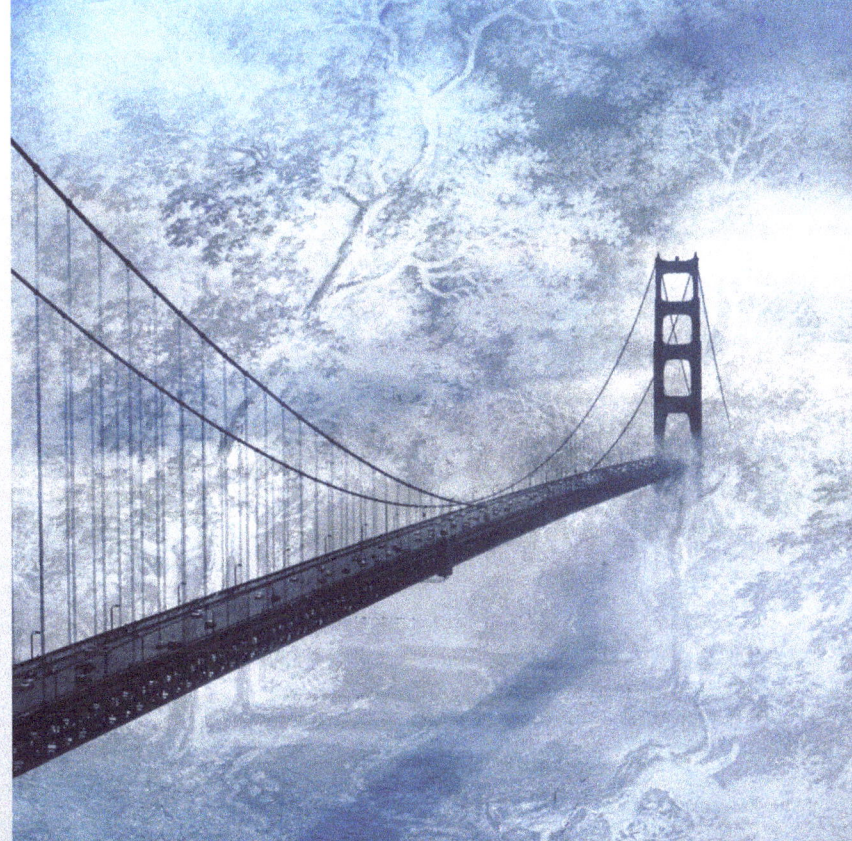

Courtesy of Carrie Shank

MAY 1

Day 121

Documentation Demand

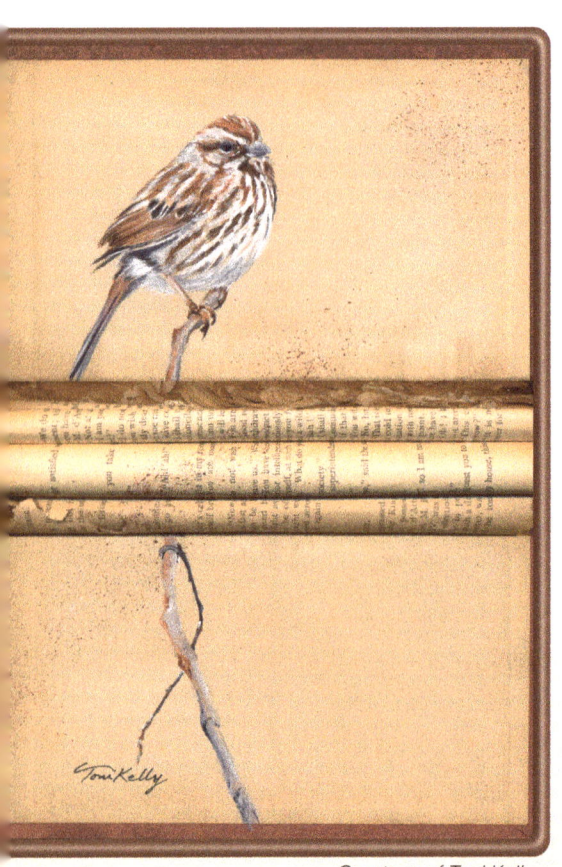
Courtesy of Toni Kelly

It is a mistake to rely only on technological advances that may reduce the time needed for clinical documentation and conducting data through an electronic health record (EHR). Residents and physicians may end up spending three times longer using the EHR as opposed to paper charting. Physicians end up spending most of their day maintaining patient health records. This not only negatively impacts job satisfaction for both residents and physicians, but it may also significantly reduce the available time needed with clients. This may have an adverse impact on patient outcomes.[130]

Today I will consider whether the document demand in my workplace results in spending more time with the computer. Time away from clients can take away the personal connection. If this is the case, can you do anything about it? How does the administration and information technology champion document demand reduction as well as having concerns about cognitive load? For every new document needing to be filled out, what documents can be taken away and rendered unnecessary? Redundant documenting can cause a lot of stress for workers when they feel conflicted between documenting demands and caring for clients. Is there an easy solution? Journal about your ideas.

May 2

Day 122

Courage to Fail

When clinical trials don't achieve desirable outcomes or when a development doesn't properly surface, researchers may lose interest. It's easier to build on positive results, which makes it simpler to secure funding for future research studies. Funding institutes generally prefer investing in hopeful projects. One could argue that research funding, resources, and time would be saved if researchers decided not to attempt experiments and studies that have already failed. However, if all failed attempts resulted in publishing new positive findings and insights, we can improve transparency and determine the best direction to take. Articles would be published more readily and built upon existing and recognized hypotheses. This, in turn, generates more useful citations and interest in medical progress.[131]

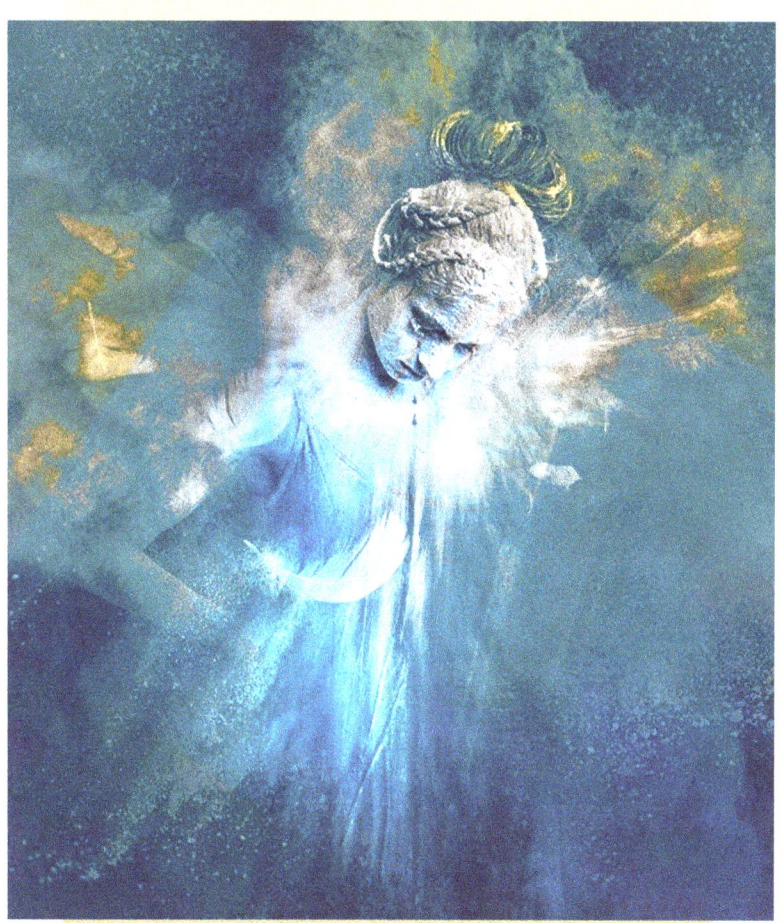

Courtesy of Carrie Shank

Today I will remember that life isn't always peaches, crème, and honey. We are human and must face challenges knowing they may lead to mistakes and failure. Having the courage to fail leads to resilience. Will you accept the negative with the positive? Brushing the negative under the rug all the time denies transparency and truth. Journal about a recent failure. What was the situation? Did you draw upon courage, and were you realistic? Did you take an optimistic approach?

MAY 3

Day 123

Communicating from the Heart

When you examine the greatest leaders of the world, you will find that they are all exceptional communicators. These leaders express their own ideas, making sure it will speak to others' aspirations and emotions. They understand that if their messages do not resonate deeply with audiences, they are likely to be misunderstood. However, it is essential to keep the mindset that communication isn't solely about you and your opinions, positions, or circumstances. It is also about assisting others through understanding and addressing their needs and concerns, and by adding actual value to their lives.[132]

Today I will consider if it is easy for me to communicate from the heart. Journal about the following. Do you sound impatient and stressed when speaking with clients, friends, or family? Has technology affected your communication in any way? Do you avoid face to face communication and hide behind a screen? Resonating with your audience and speaking from your heart is a learned talent. However, what are the positions, circumstances, and opinions of others? Adding value to other's lives is what matters when you communicate from the heart.

Courtesy of Jill Santi

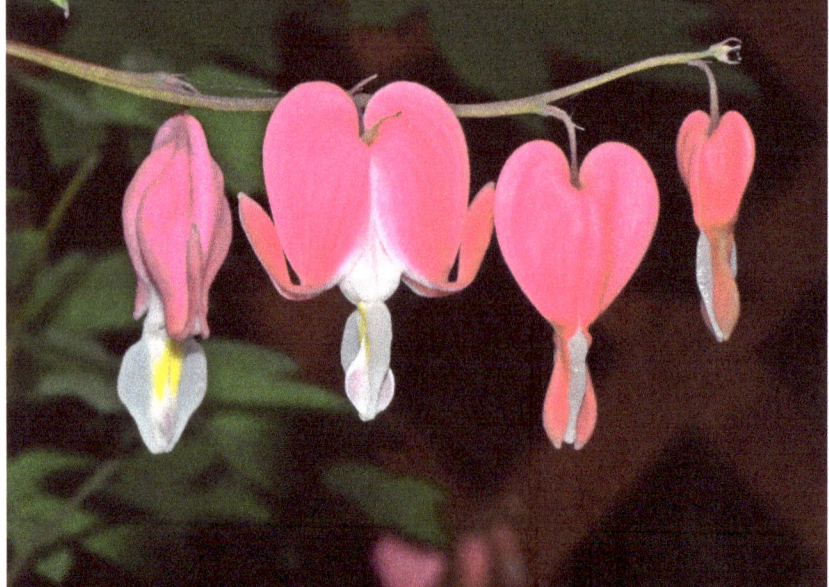

MAY 4

Day 124

Morale

It is unfortunate that many managers tend not to care about employee morale. Instead, they often push and prod through any necessary means. Managers may fail to comprehend that they have a huge impact on the overall effectiveness of the company. They have a major influence on the bottom line, productivity, and ability for a company to retain its talent.[133]

Today I will observe the morale in my workplace. In your journal, on a scale of 1-10, how would you rate the morale, with 10 being the most positive and 1 being the least positive? What number do you rate your workplace? If the number is low, can you think of a few reasons why? Is the reason because of the manager, or the messages the manager delivers from above? What do organizations at the unit level do to improve morale? Can you name a few things your workplace does to build self-esteem and confidence? Is your workplace retaining staff due to a high rating of morale?

Courtesy of Toni Kelly

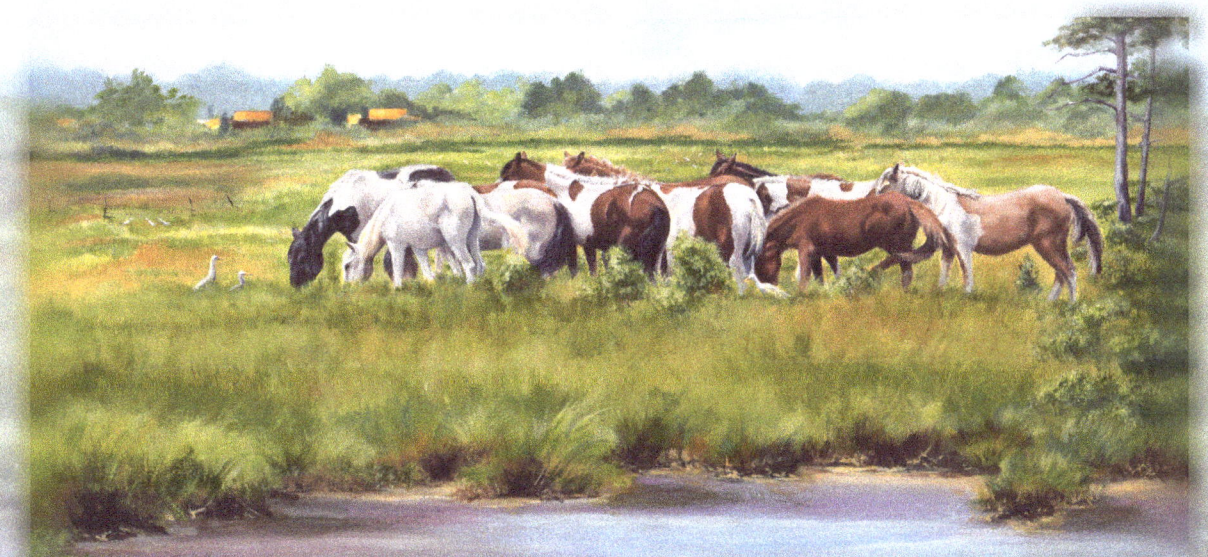

MAY 5

Day 125

Pessimism

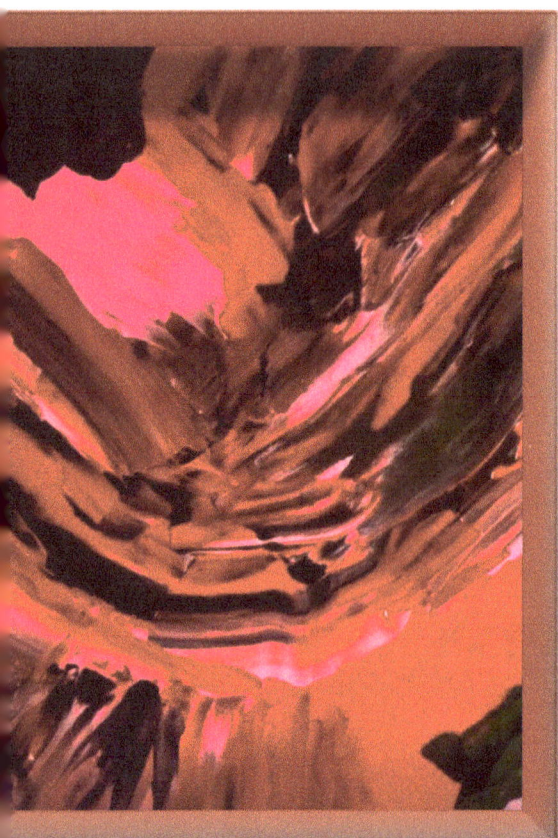

Courtesy of Aryn Grayson

Depending on your outlook, you can view the glass as being half-empty or half-full. Which way does your viewpoint lean when you get out of bed most mornings? Do you feel that optimism or pessimism can truly impact your health? It has been a question contemplated throughout decades, and this issue has sparked a huge interest in the self-help genre. Directing your focus toward staying positive, especially when you face something devastating, such as a serious illness, is key. Scientific evidence supporting a sunny outlook is controversial, contradictory, and contentious. For instance, when there are higher levels of pessimism present, there is a link to inflammation and cardiac death. However, optimistic or pessimistic personality traits showing a link to cardiac disease and death are scarce. Therefore, understand that studies may point toward an association, not necessarily to a "cause and effect." There are no studies that prove that pessimism can cause a person to die prematurely.[134]

Today I will remember that even though being pessimistic most likely won't kill me, people do not respond to complaining. How can you express yourself in a neutral or positive way? Journal about how you can try to be a bit more optimistic, have hope, or perhaps believe that something wonderful is around the corner. Being chained to a pessimistic spirit has its risks and may contribute to serious illness. How do you get out of bed most mornings? Is your glass half-full? Do you turn lemons into lemonade?

MAY 6

Day 126

Overly Optimistic

Having a positive attitude is good, but when you are overly optimistic, it's possible to lose touch with reality.

- Over-optimism leads to overconfidence and impracticality.
- Thoughts about what may go wrong lead to prevention.
- Mental strength is produced with a balance between optimism and realism.
- Reality is built by developing comfort with the truth.[135]

Today I will remember to be realistic and optimistic. Do you consider yourself overly optimistic? Having a good balance of optimism and realism builds mental muscle, confidence, and practicality. Journal about the things you are doing to stay positive. Planning and prevention are logical ways to build confidence.

Courtesy of Rachel Brown

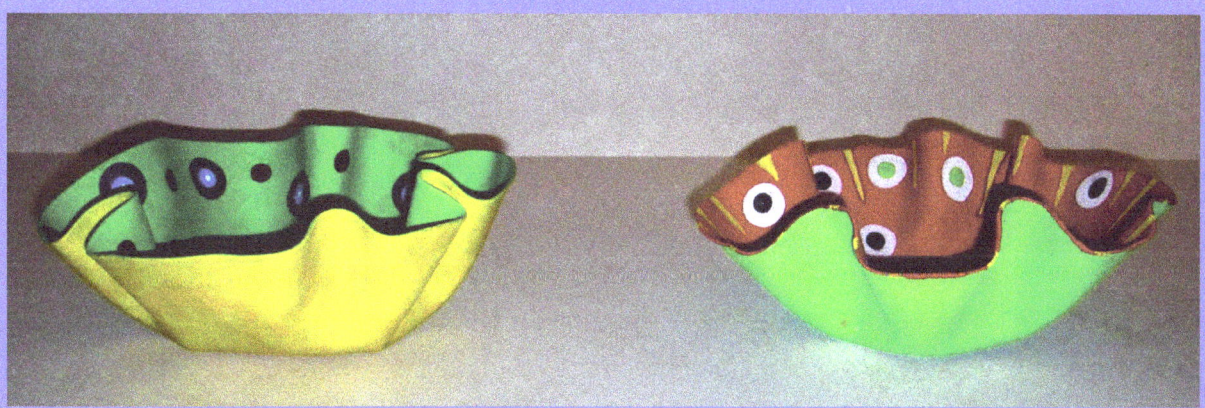

MAY 7

Day 127

New Challenges

Tackling new challenges helps prove dedication, a good work ethic, and the capability of leading your organization toward success. However, these additional responsibilities can also be overwhelming and stressful. Before accepting new roles within your company, you need to reflect upon whether your work and life will be balanced to make certain it is the proper fit for you.[136]

Today I will consider not taking on more than I can handle when given a choice. Journal about new challenges at work that can make things better for your organization, and about the impact additional responsibilities could have on you. Exhaustion, stress, and work-life imbalance are just a few things to evaluate. Be mindful of the challenges you choose.

Courtesy of Charles Freedom Long

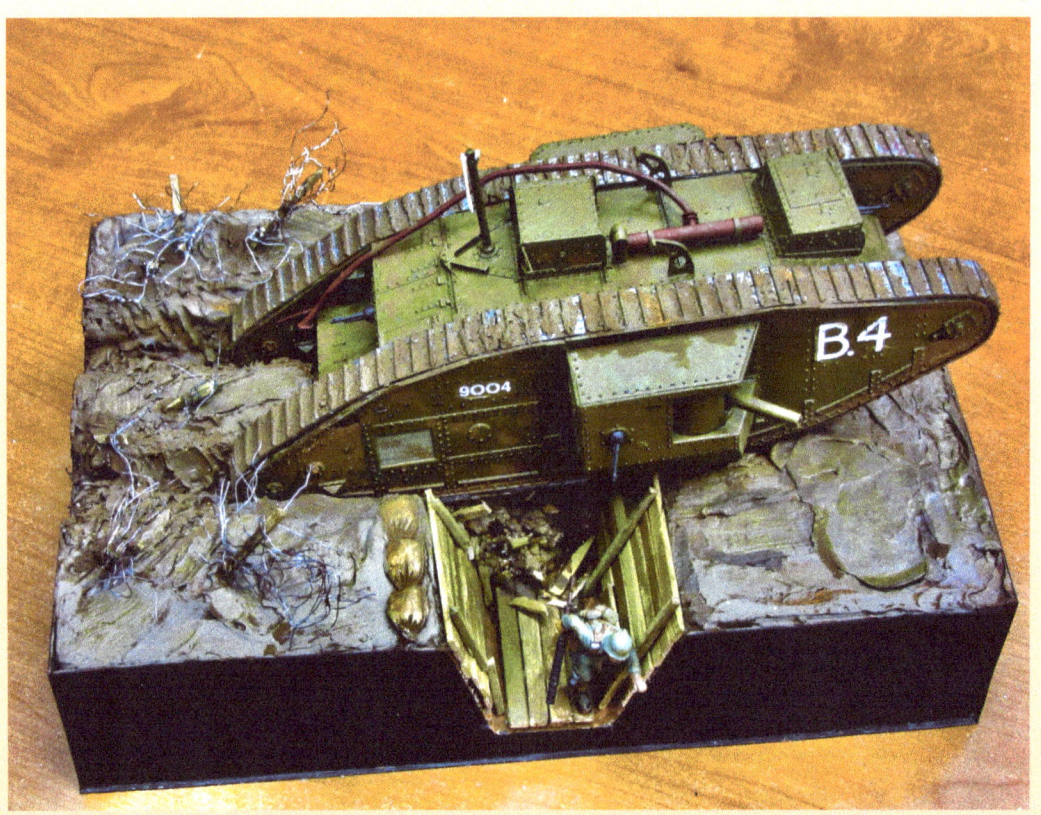

MAY 8

Day 128

Blame

Disturbing stories have been reported by clinicians suggesting the concept of resilience is used by employers to narrow in on employees' failures instead of investigating the wider aspects of the practice. Clinicians state that resilience is often used to distract attention from system failures, resulting from significant concerns like cuts in funding along with "workforce churn." Although limited, findings indicated an alarming trend that blamed the workers for their stress, burnout, and failure to cope. This was a way of placing the focus of change on the workers. However, without considering broader issues, it is dangerous to ascribe culpability towards "non-resilient workers" or blaming them for the troubles of their own making. Research suggests that employers may have limited comprehension of the interconnected and complex organizational structures, along with individual ability. For some, the concept of resilience results in an increased blame culture.[137]

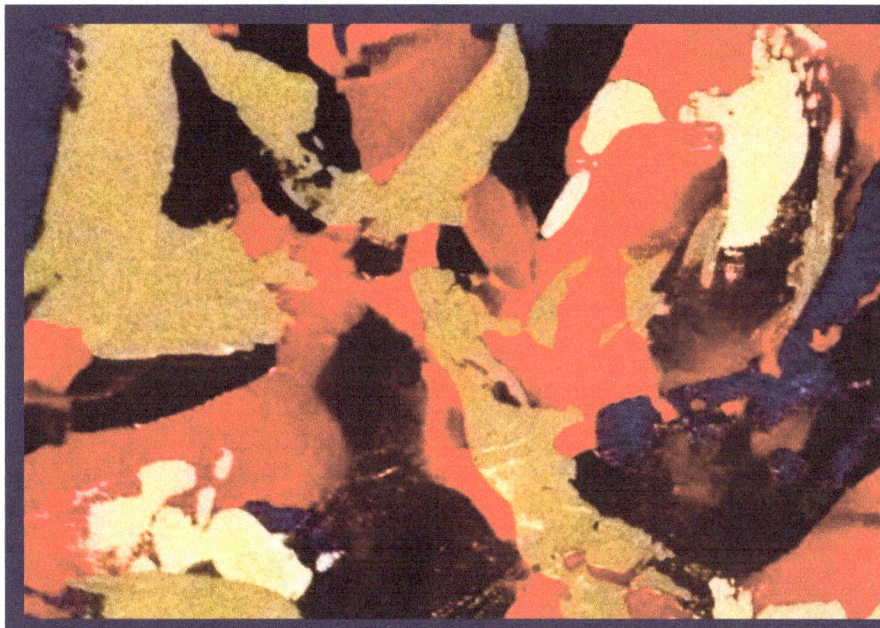

Courtesy of Aryn Grayson

Today I will consider that I am already resilient and don't necessarily need more training in resilience. I realize that organizations need to fix the systems so that employees are not overworked or overly stressed. Journal about how system issues, technology, documentation overload, or endless new quality endeavors can create more work and lead to burnout within your workplace. How can you stop blaming yourself and others for burnout and start pointing the finger of blame where it should be, at systems that do not fund properly or have the right resources?

MAY 9

Day 129

Taking a Vacation

Many studies report that taking time off from work on occasion can contribute to both physical and psychological health benefits. Those taking a vacation tend to show lower signs of stress, have a lower risk of heart disease, have a more positive outlook toward life, and have more motivation for achieving goals.[138]

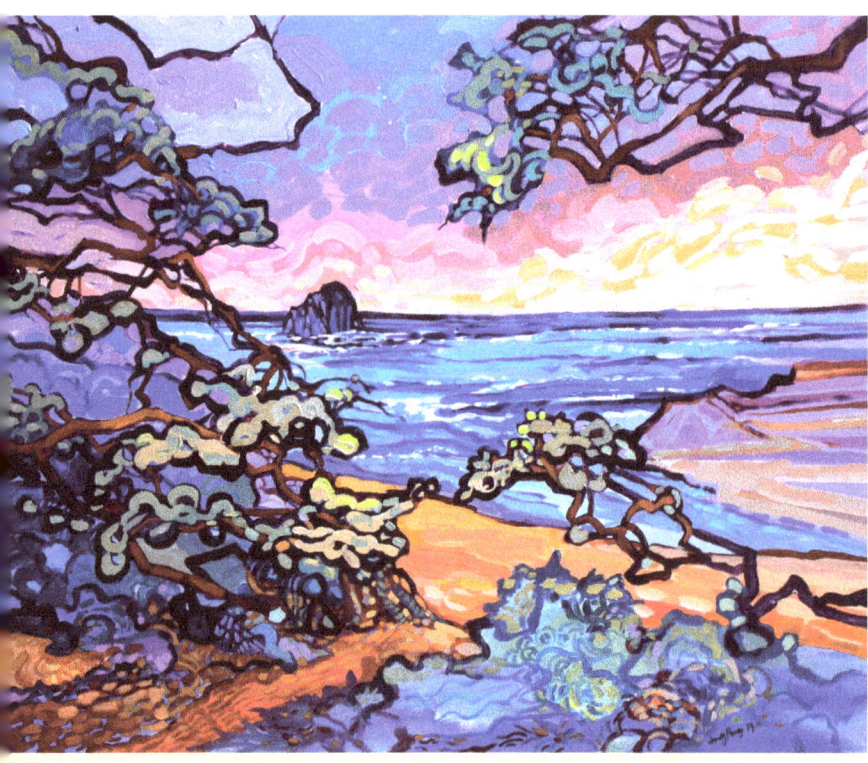

Courtesy of Judy Hodge

Today I am going to plan a vacation. Whether it is a long weekend or a two-week vacation, any time away from work is wonderful and healthy. Start a self-care goal while on vacation. Start small with just 10 minutes of deep breathing exercises each day. Journal about where you would like to go and what you would like to do while on vacation in order to clear your mind. Do it now. Prevent your burnout.

MAY 10
Day 130

Authentic Self

We seek our authentic self from within. We search through desires, emotions, thoughts, and behaviors wanting manifestation. We can never find our authentic self from someone else's opinion, cultural or social belief system, family agenda, social mores, or external sources. We only locate it by reflecting within. The authentic self tries to find small ways of presenting itself. It wants a peaceful, congruent relationship with us. Each day, the authentic self wants to show us how to become our true self. It wants to reveal our authentic, original thoughts, beliefs, genuine behaviors, and feelings.[139]

Today I will think about my authentic self. I will consider what is important to me, my thoughts, what I believe in, what I feel, and how I behave. What matters is my authentic self, not pretending to be someone just to make other people happy. Think about how pretending to be someone that you are not can wear you down. Does it create stress and exhaustion, both emotionally and spiritually? Do you see how that could lead to burnout? Being genuine begins in your own mindset. Be yourself today and each day. Journal about authentic self.

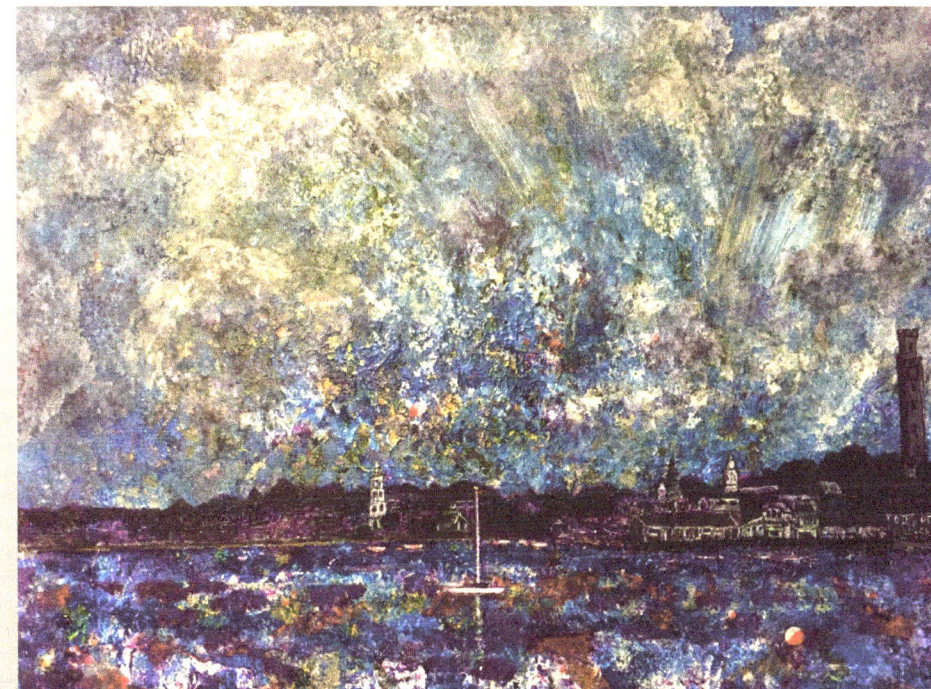

Courtesy of Peter Sterling Turner

MAY 11

Day 131

Stamina

Stamina is defined as the energy and strength used to preserve mental or physical effort over extended periods. By improving your stamina, you are helping yourself decrease discomfort or stress during activities. You are also reducing symptoms of fatigue and exhaustion. Greater stamina enables daily activities to be performed at a higher level while consuming less energy.[140]

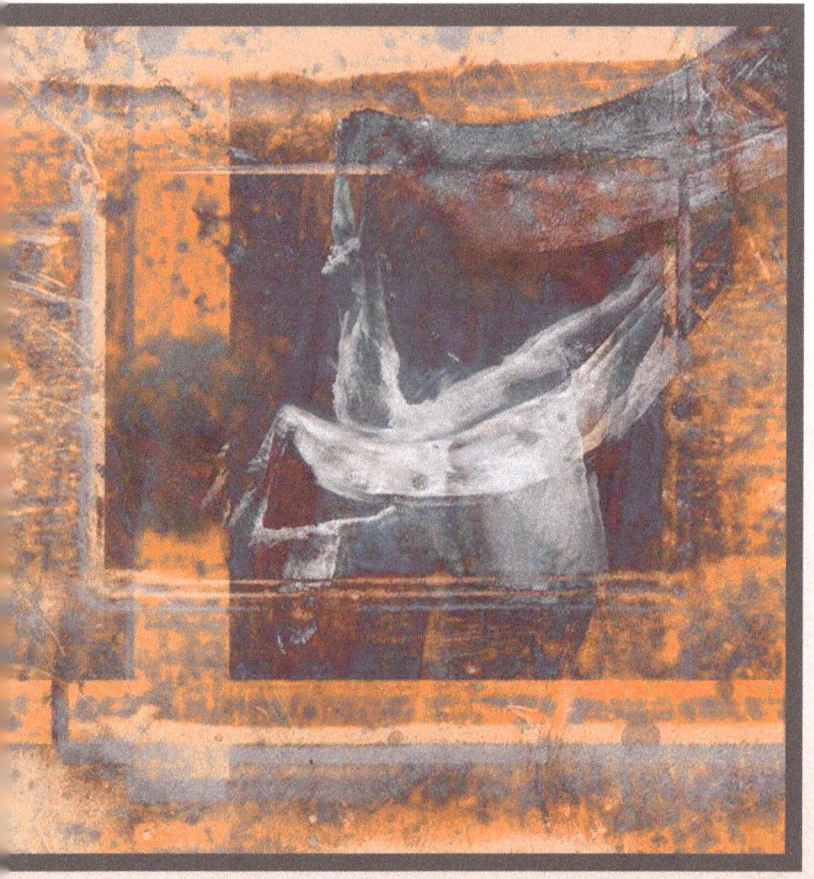

Courtesy of Carrie Shank

Today I will evaluate my stamina. Rate yourself as either being weak, moderately strong, or the strongest. Evaluate yourself both physically and mentally. Do you listen to yourself when your stamina is low, and you need to rest? Do you listen to yourself when you need to expel more energy and are feeling particularly strong? Journal about how taking time to reflect on stamina can be helpful in planning and preventing exhaustion. What three things can you do to gain more stamina? Make a list.

Excellence

Worrying about mistakes can turn life into a punishing perfection pursuit. A prerequisite of perfectionism is having concerns over doubts, actions, and mistakes. Obsessed that failure will lead others to have bad thoughts about them, perfectionists seem to have an intrinsic performance self-evaluation. Perfectionists are haunted by the opinions of colleagues and superiors over task completion and have a reluctance to acknowledge something as being finished. We are always striving for accuracy within our work, and this is a way of seeking excellence. Think about nurses or doctors as they are administering medications to their clients. Accuracy is not the same as perfection. A person who directs their focus on excellence takes pride in having 100% accuracy when providing medication to clients. Those who focus on perfectionism deliver similar 100% accuracy, but they are hung up on whether they did it perfectly correct.[141]

Today I will consider if I am practicing excellence or perfectionism. Understand how stress-inducing that is for you. True, many of us in our work and life must have precision and 100% accuracy, but that doesn't necessarily mean that you are a perfectionist. Being accurate, precise, and exhibiting excellence at work is very different from neurotic perfectionism. Journal about whether perfectionism introduces stress into your daily life or how you are able to focus on excellence instead.

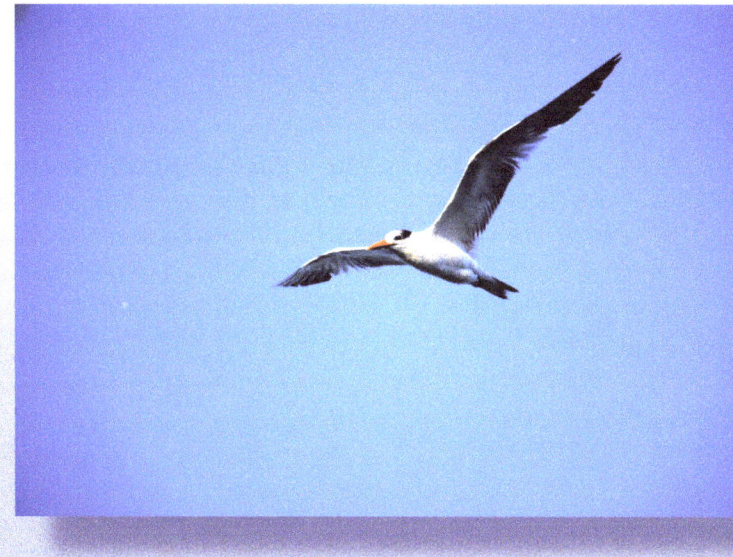

Courtesy of Linda Probst

MAY 13
Day 133

Perseverance

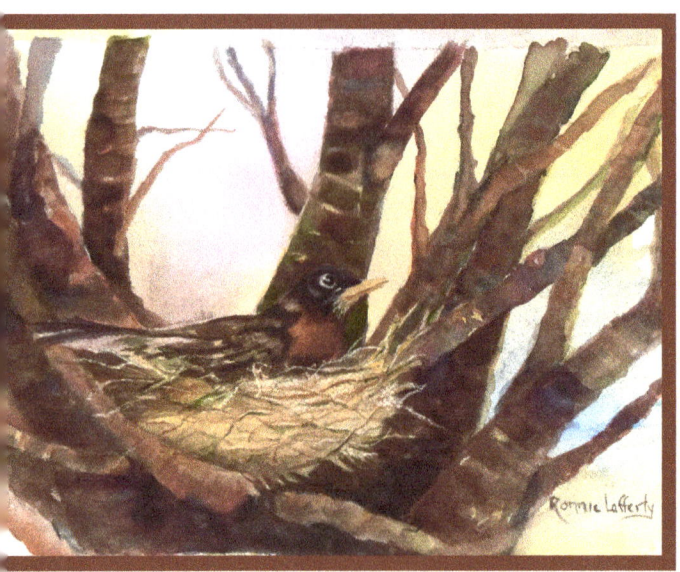
Courtesy of Ronnie Lafferty

An emotionally draining work environment inevitably has negative effects on businesses. In disruptive market situations, CEOs often will face many different pressures. For example, the expectation of adapting to altering trends within the workplace or retaining talent. This results in burnout for CEOs and is just as apparent as burnout in employees. Leaders must remember to slow down thinking to detach from their emotions, which are in an autopilot state produced by stressful environments. They must learn to recognize and manage perseverance in their employees.[142]

Today I will consider if I am emotionally drained from my job. We really need to discuss perseverance as a work skill. The landscape is similar in many professions. The common factors are exhaustion, work overload, stress, cynicism, and depersonalization, leading to burnout. In your journal, what plans do you have for burnout prevention for yourself? Being able to persevere under high-pressure environments takes tenacity and resilience.

MAY 14

Day 134

Being Mindful

In a well-known study, Moody (2013) and colleagues spent eight weeks studying and learning about practicing mindfulness. The study included social workers, nurses, psychologists, and physicians who cared for pediatric cancer patients at hospitals in Israel and the United States. Questionnaires that researchers administered following the completion of their study demonstrated that intervention didn't reduce staff level of burnout, stress, or depression. However, data within diaries that the caregivers used during the course showed that intervention did result in positive effects. Staff reported in their journals that the course brought an increased sense of inner peace and helped decrease stress and anxiety. By using the tools in the course, staff learned abilities to relax their minds and let go of negative thinking. The course also prepared them to better finesse stressful situations, such as giving a diagnosis to a patient and their family. Staff also indicated their increase in the awareness of their actions and thoughts, which helped them become more efficient in their work, and better at focusing on their goals. Being mindful helped the staff feel proud of their work since they could reflect upon their behaviors and truly appreciate the effects.[143]

Today I will consider the effects of journaling. Journaling helps make you aware of your thoughts and behaviors. When you are aware, you are mindful. Up to this point in the workbook, evaluate whether journaling is helping you. Reread your journal thus far. Does journaling help you relax and let go of anxiety or stress? What have you experienced while using your Healing Burnout Guide journal? Do you feel more mindful?

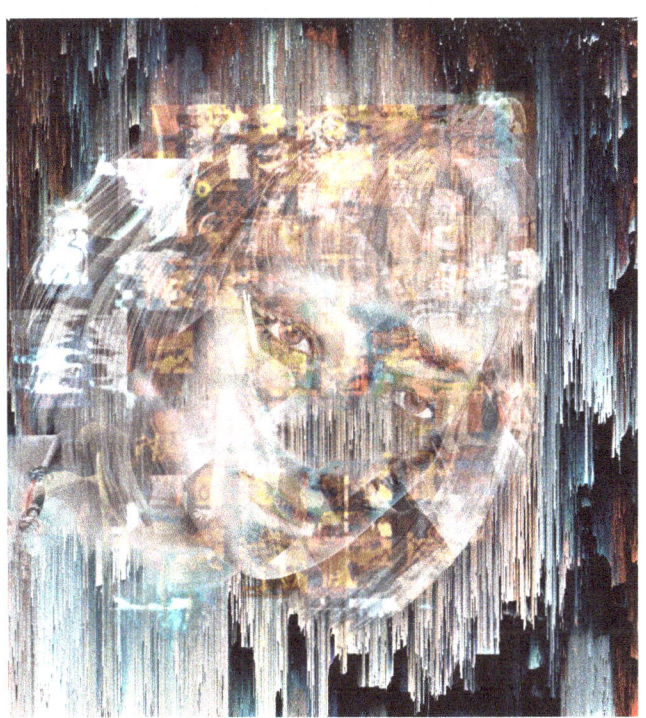

Courtesy of Carrie Shank

MAY 15
Day 135

Write it Down

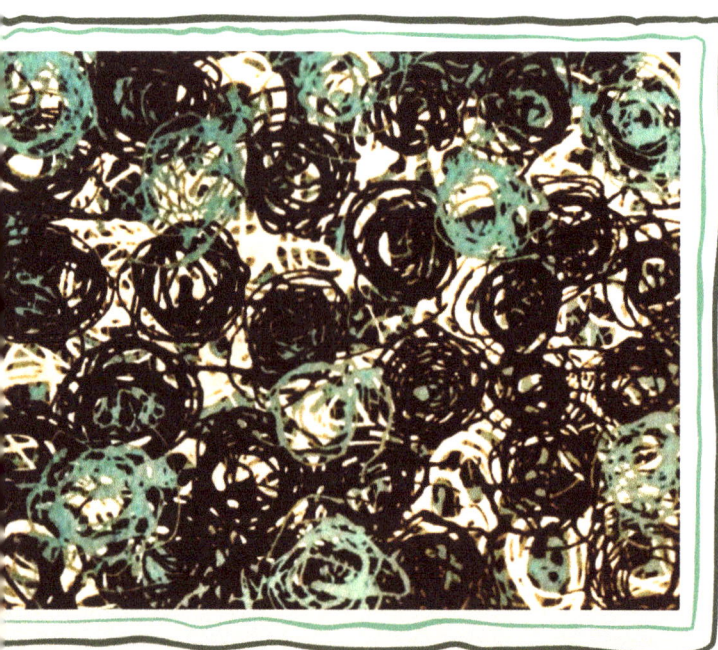

Courtesy of Aryn Grayson

Today I will consider how writing things down can help reduce disorganization and stress. When there is clutter in an overactive mind, it can help to write a list and check things off as you accomplish them. Instead of memorizing mental lists, the act of writing them down relieves tension and stress. Make a list in your journal now of the things you need to get done. Notice the sensation once the list is created. Try it.

Writing down a list is an excellent way of clearing your mind. When you write down your thoughts, you'll start to feel relieved, like a weight lifting off your back. Even before you tackle the list, you will feel a sense of transformation where your brain begins to move from chaos into the first stages of becoming organized. You will have a visual list of your plans, goals, and thoughts without having to rely solely on memory. Itemize everything that is on your mind. You may notice that when you are ruminating about everything, you feel stressed. In turn, it can cause you to be unproductive. We often become crippled by unconscious thoughts about all the things we do wrong, resulting in feeling unfulfilled. Sadly, we may repeat daily cycles of rumination. To solve this issue effectively, write it down! It may seem like an unnecessary step; however, it has been significantly and scientifically proven that writing down thoughts that haunt us can turn chaos into simplicity.[144]

MAY 16

Day 136

Socially Aware

Gambs (1942), a professor at Louisiana State University, wrote about the meaning of social awareness. He thought that being socially aware meant knowing, in every particle and fiber of our body, a psychological principle that people have significance only as part of a group. Men and women can be successful only when giving themselves generously and freely to a group. When we lose ourselves, we find ourselves. When we love others, we receive their love. "By living for others - and dying if need be - we achieve immortality." When socially aware, we understand applications and ramifications with the importance in families, classrooms, social and economic concerns, and international diplomacy.[145]

Today I will consider the group that I belong to at work. I will think about each member and what they may be going through at work or home. Journal about the following. How can you be helpful to them? Is there anything you can give, whether it is time, assistance, advice, support, or just listening? When you consider others around you in your group, you begin to be socially aware. When you have a supportive social group, you feel like you belong, which can alleviate a lot of stress at work.

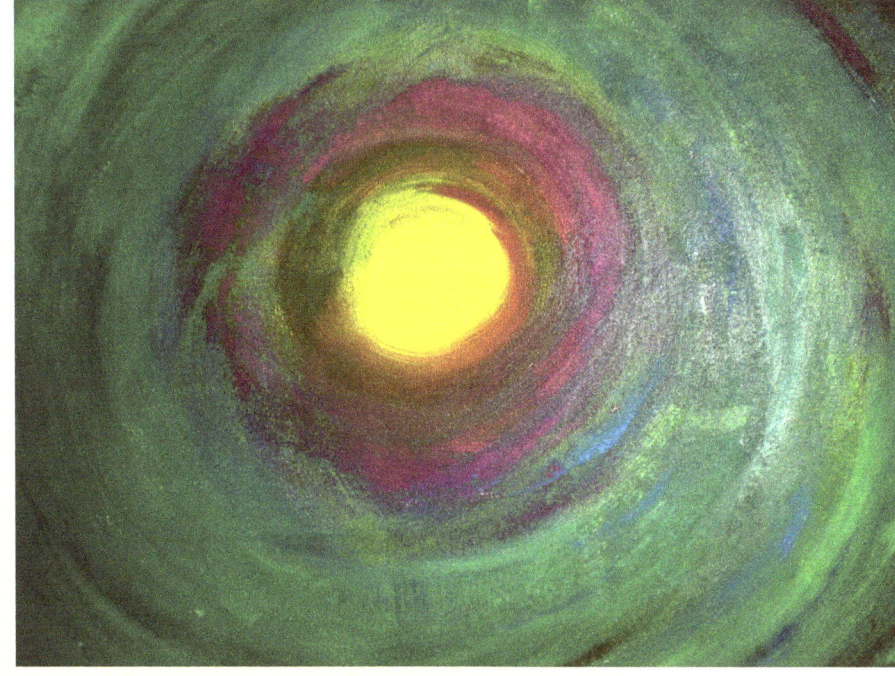

Courtesy of Peter Sterling Turner

MAY 17

Day 137

Mood

Moods have a connection with stories we have told ourselves about "how things are," as well as our rendering of what surrounds us. Our perception and handling of moods will either open us or close us to opportunities and possibilities. Additionally, moods may have either a negative or positive impact on our wellbeing, bodies, and overall health. Our moods may spread to others around us. You have likely witnessed within your work environment when one coworker shows up after waking up on the "wrong side of the bed." By the afternoon, the entire team seems to be grouchy. Our moods, both negative and positive, can also be contagious within communities.[146] Defining mood can also be challenging since one person's judgment will depend on their perception of moods in another. Mood is a "highly subjective concept." Diverse personalities and emotional tones are a way of expressing your mood.[147]

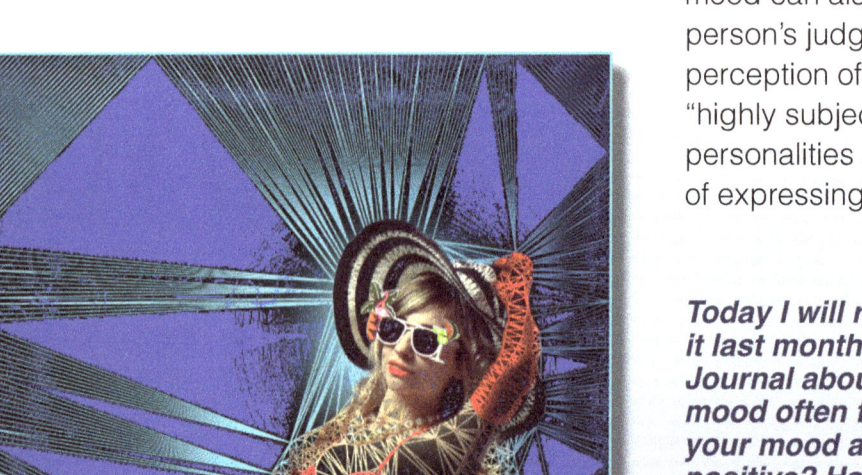

Courtesy of Carrie Shank

Today I will reflect on my mood. How was it last month, last week, and today? Journal about the following. Does your mood often fluctuate? Would you rate your mood as usually negative or positive? Have you perhaps mistaken someone's mood at work as toxic? Were they instead exhausted, stressed, experiencing depersonalization, or maybe burned out? What caused the bad mood? Were they being overworked, ignored, or was there something happening at home?

MAY 18

Day 138

Thriving

People can fluctuate between three different states of struggling, thriving, or illness. Those with a significant mental health concern can thrive at work with the right amount of support. For that to be possible, people must have a quality working environment that is principled with fair pay, autonomy, a healthy work-life balance, and opportunities to advance. Their work must also be absent from harassment and bullying. When the proper conditions and needs are met, it may prevent any additional mental health problems from arising. Supporting people that have existing conditions to excel at their work is possible.[148]

Today I will evaluate my workplace and whether it offers autonomy, fair pay, a good work-life balance, and opportunities to advance. If these conditions are not present in the workplace, what kind of environment are you in? Do harassment and bullying exist in your workplace? If so, are there opportunities to improve it? Evaluate each good work principle. What things does your workplace do to support the mental health of employees? Are you thriving or struggling? What's YOUR plan to thrive?

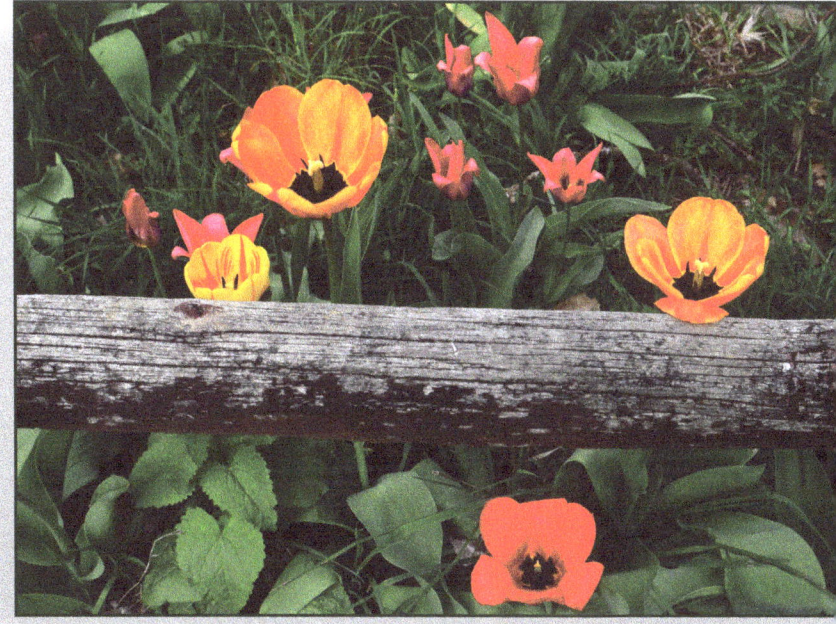

Courtesy of Jill Santi

MAY 19

Day 139

Constant Changes

Healthcare systems are complex, adaptive, and filled with constant changes. The performance and behaviors change with time. Understanding the individual components of healthcare isn't simple. Compared to other systems such as the military, manufacturing, education, or banking – healthcare remains the most complex. There's a wide range of moving parts within the healthcare industry that caters to clients with diverse needs and several options or interventions compared with other sectors. Because of the clients' individual needs and uncertain presentations, there exist multiple clinically focused processes. There are numerous stakeholders within healthcare, having various interests and differing roles while heavily regulated controls are in place. There are endless combinations of events, activities, interactions, and outcomes.[149]

Today I will consider how adaptable I am to change. Do constant changes irritate you? Be truthful. Just when you get used to one way of doing something, someone has a bright idea to change the workflow or process another way. This can be disruptive to workers and cause stress. What choice do you have in the work that affects you? Sometimes change is good, but not when you're changing only for the sake of changing. For every new change implemented, there may be a positive result or unintended consequences. Select your changes carefully. Journal about any recent changes you went through and how you reacted?

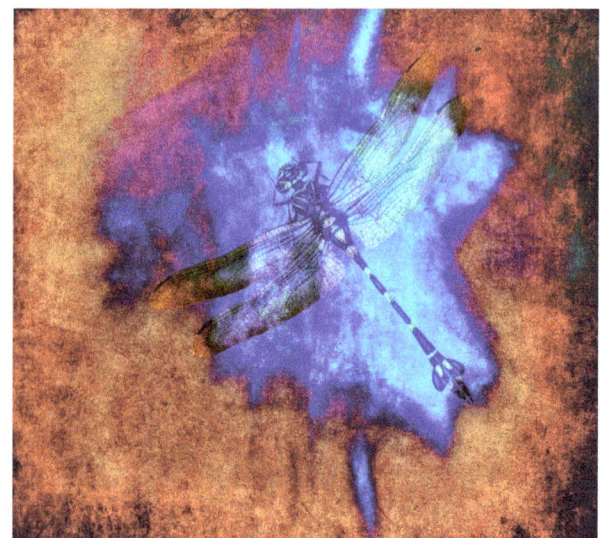

Courtesy of Carrie Shank

MAY 20
Day 140

Firmly Grounded

Grounding unites us with the present. It helps pull us into the physical encounter of the moment. It can create a sensation of ease within the mind and balance within the body. Grounding generates calm, alleviates stress, and prompts us to recall who we really are by redirecting our attention to help us feel more at home within our bodies. A fantastic way to become and stay grounded is to practice yoga asana. It focuses on our breath and body. It is a sound way to experience self-awareness. Each yoga pose supports grounding.

Try these poses:
- Marjaryasana/Bitilasana (Cat/Cow pose)
- Tadasana (Mountain pose)
- Utkatasana (Chair pose)
- Savasana (Corpse pose)
- Utkata Konasana (Goddess pose)[150]

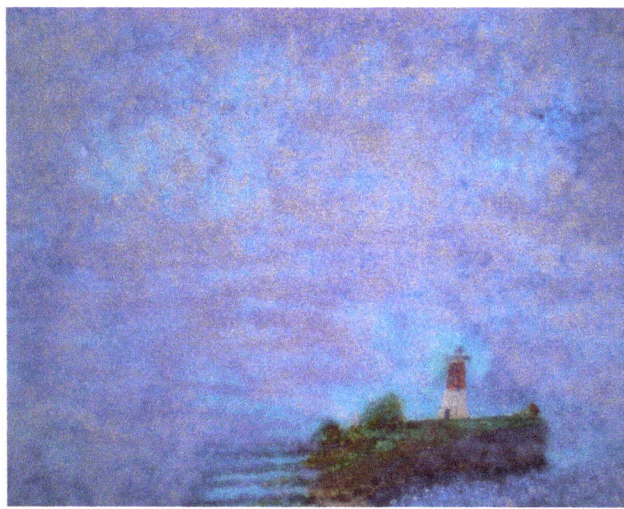

Courtesy of Peter Sterling Turner

Today I will consider becoming more grounded with a yoga practice. Some yoga poses could be incorporated into your workday for on the spot grounding when tension begins to build because of irritations, unplanned changes, or just annoying nuisances. When your mood is disrupted, and you feel stressed out, another easy grounding exercise is Nadi Shodhana Pranayama: Alternate Nostril Breathing,[151] which doesn't require leaving your chair. Journal about which poses you have tried and which have proven to be most helpful to you.

Day 141

MAY 21

Serving Others

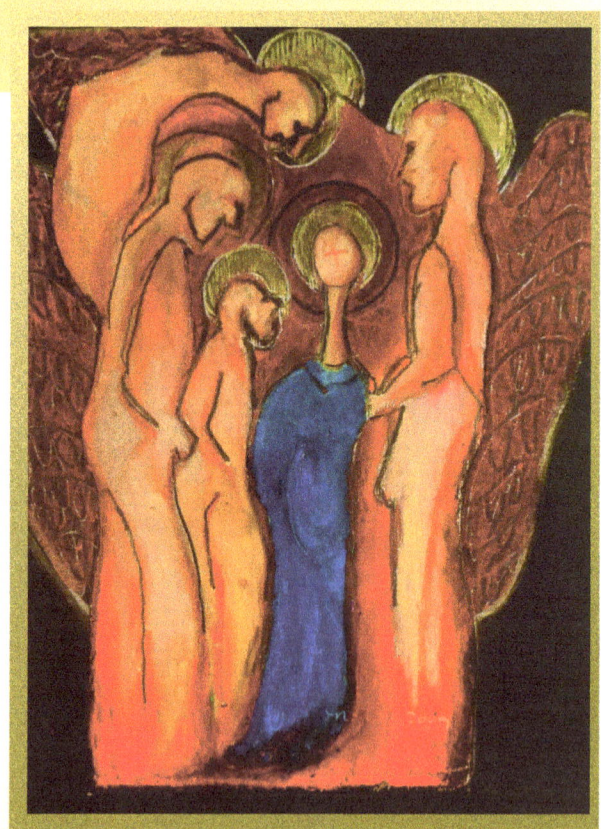

Courtesy of Nancy Nixon Ensign

We live in a very stressful world in which healthcare workers suffer tremendously from burnout that is painful and slow. Many that work long hours while raising their families may be reaching burnout also. Many feel they are very exhausted from giving to others, although giving is a main source of joy in their lives. Giving to others and forming connections in positive ways brings long-lasting feelings of happiness that come from living with meaning and a purpose.[152]

Today, I will reflect on serving others and my giving habits. Do you give more than you receive? Do you receive more than you give? When you are exhausted and overworked, how easy is giving? Think about a time when you just didn't have it in you to give more, but you did anyway. In your journal, describe the situation. You may find more joy in life by serving others, but don't forget to take care of yourself.

MAY 22
Day 142

Professional Development

Within the always growing and changing education sector, individual success has become quite a challenge for leading society. There are demands placed on academicians for improving their professional careers and achieving degrees for their promotions. Academics are required to increase their professional development by obtaining more knowledge and skills while supporting coworkers and students. Educational development is a key factor that allows for the potential of a society. Faculty are required to meet with parents, their students, administrative and other staff, leading to stress and burnout. Also, academics desire quality teaching and outstanding levels of success. Another reason for stress and burnout of teachers, professors, and faculty is their responsibilities for student performance in addition to their own professional development and achievement. Academicians may be dissatisfied with their jobs, feel exhausted, and feel like quitting, especially when there are performance and administrative pressures.[153]

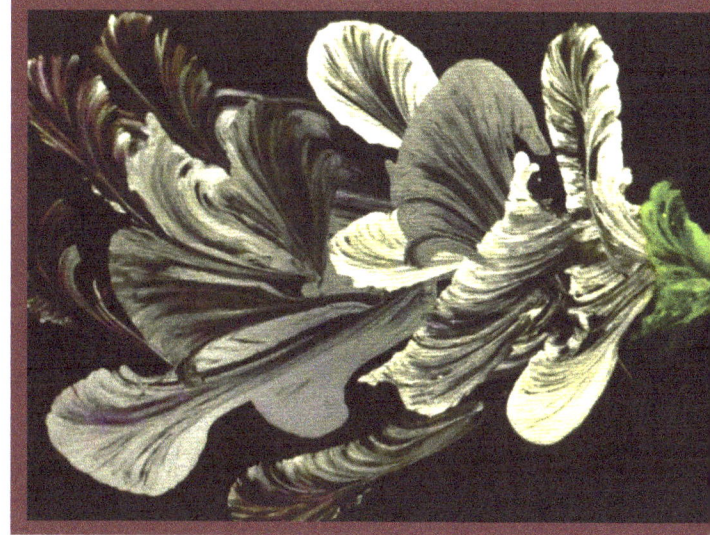

Courtesy of Aryn Grayson

Today I will consider the pressure I am under to deliver outstanding outcomes. While professional development generally is how one develops their expertise, the pressure to do so creates a lot of stress, exhaustion, and burned out academics forced to "publish or perish." This kind of climate and normalizing burnout is not conducive to health and healing. Journal about whether professional development has caused any pressure, stress, or burnout for you.

MAY 23
Day 143

Involvement in Decision-Making

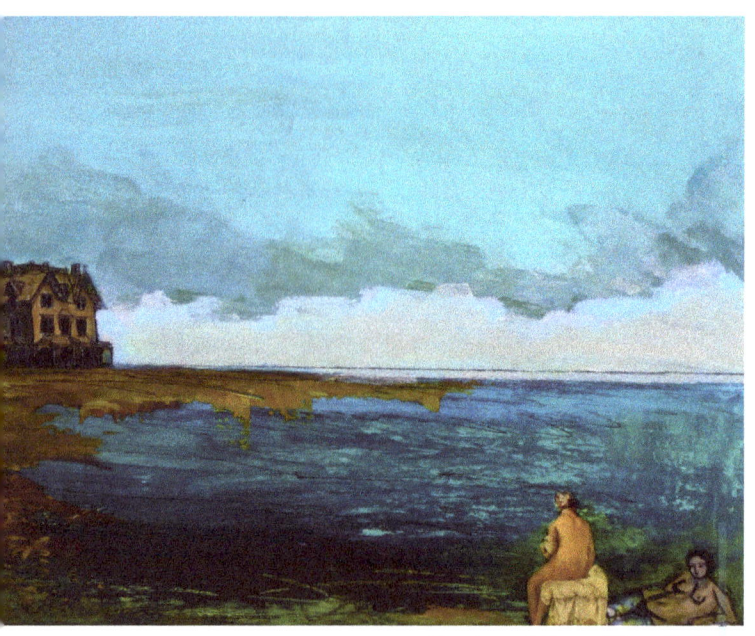
Courtesy of Nancy Nixon Ensign

People are a solid foundation for any successful company. Employees represent the ideas and knowledge behind a company, yet too often, are an untapped resource. It is important that workers have involvement in decision-making processes. This not only allows for contribution to the successes within an organization, but it can also save companies both money and time through an increase in productivity and reduction in outsourcing. As functioning participants in decision-making processes, employees realize their ideas can be important contributions to their companies. In turn, this gives them the power to influence outcomes in the work they do, which leads to increased job satisfaction and more positive attitudes toward both their positions and the company.[154]

Today evaluate whether your company allows you to participate in decision-making, at least involving the work that you do. Journal about the following. Are there opportunities for you to be part of committees or councils at work? Do you and your coworkers contribute to decision-making processes within your company? When everything is handed top-down with no staff involvement, it makes for an environment with less employee satisfaction, which can lead to stress and negativity within the workplace.

MAY 24

Day 144

Realistic Optimism

Realistic optimists understand the need for thinking mindfully. When they can be prepared and stay organized, they become more aware of the risks involved with mitigation plans. This state of mind can stimulate confidence levels, leading to increased optimistic outlooks toward success rates. Understanding how to be both optimistic yet realistic simultaneously may help people remain calm, especially during periods of crisis.[155]

Today I will consider if I have developed a realistic optimism over time. Assess your confidence level. Journal about how realistic optimism in times of crisis may help you feel organized, prepared, and calm. Describe a time when you needed to remain calm, and your optimism helped you stay confident and mindful.

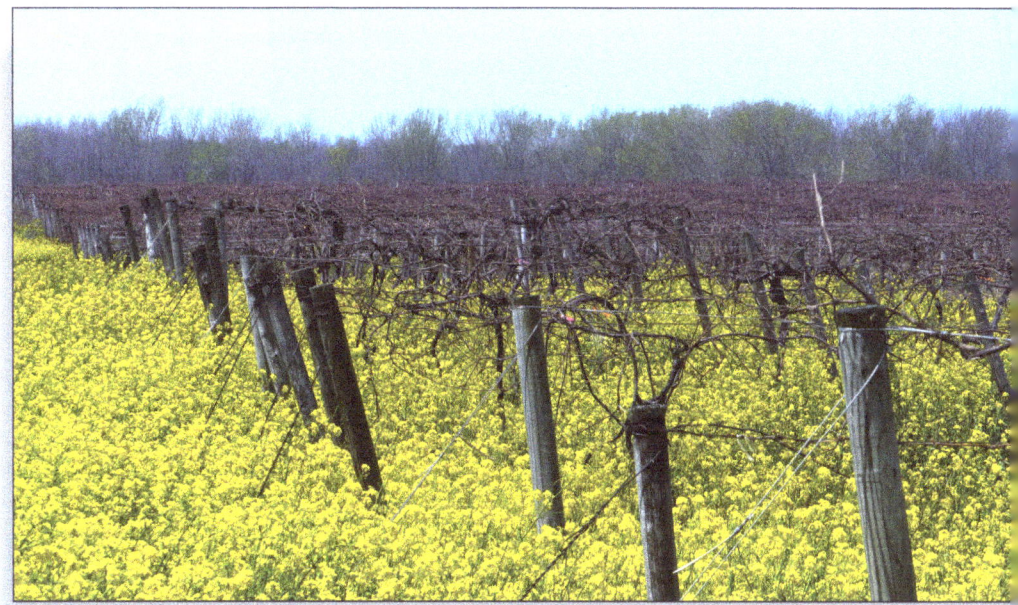

Courtesy of Spar Ki

Day 145

MAY 25

Talking with your Boss

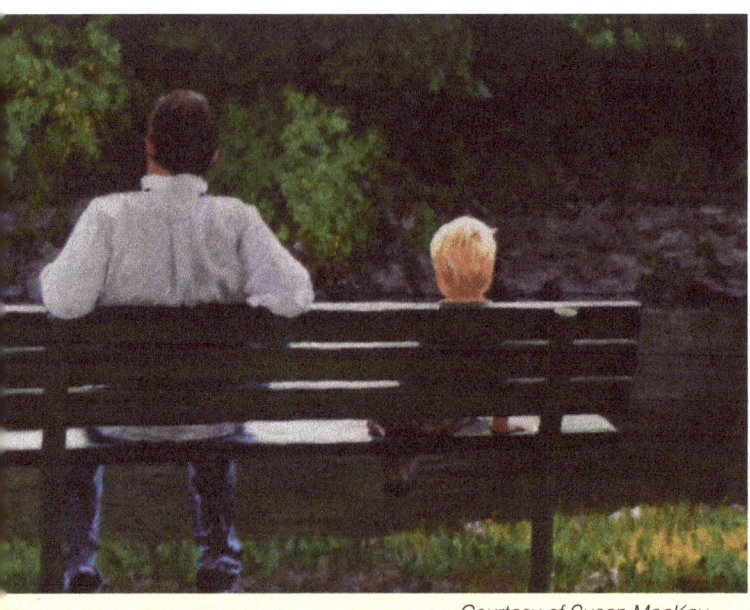
Courtesy of Susan MacKay

When talking with your boss, try to avoid rambling stories, lengthy speeches, and drawn-out preambles. Once you are known for being unnecessarily verbose or too time-draining, your boss may start to purposely avoid you, which may ruin your relationship. When it's possible, try cutting directly to the chase with the exact information you want to share. Doing this will hopefully encourage your boss to do the same with you.[156]

Today I will consider the relationship I have with my boss. Is your boss a "boss," or are they a "leader" that you can follow? Try to keep your communications professional and relevant with your "boss." Look up "best tips for talking with your boss." Journal about the last conversation you had. Do you have similar or different communication styles? Sometimes less is more, especially with a "boss."

MAY 26

Day 146

Validate Yourself

Courtesy of Carrie Shank

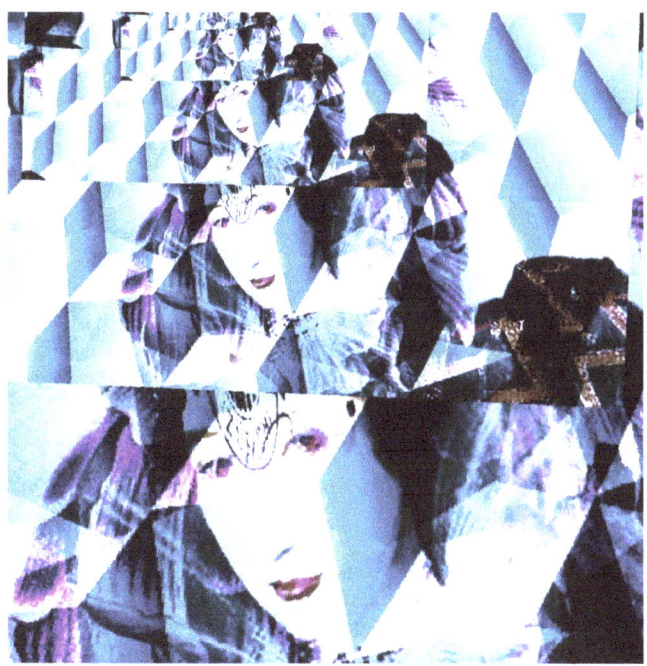

Today I will validate myself. What you are thinking and feeling is real, and it matters. You are not wrong for these thoughts or feelings. They are just what they are, thoughts and feelings. You are not imagining these emotions; they are really yours. Sometimes we do not want to suffer the consequences of revealing our position on an issue. Give yourself permission to validate yourself today and each day. Write about the last time you validated yourself. What was the situation? What holds you back from validation?

Self-validation is the acceptance of your internal thoughts, experiences, and feelings. Self-validation doesn't mean believing your feelings and thoughts are legitimate. You will often think thoughts that may shock you or not mirror your values or what you believe to be true. You may also experience feelings that are not justified. Fighting these feelings and thoughts or judging yourself when you have them increases emotional distress. You may also lose out on valuable information about you as a whole person. Through validation of your emotions and thoughts, you can be calm and cope more productively. Validating yourself can help you better understand and accept yourself, which will lead to an identity that is stronger and ability to improve skills at managing difficult emotions. Self-validation can help you discover wisdom.[157]

MAY 27
Day 147

Doing Great Work

Work often seems bureaucratic, which can be mentally exhausting. Doing good work entails being effective and satisfying your job requirements. Good work is important, but doing great work is what matters most. Great work has more meaning and makes a stronger impact. Employees and organizations are expected to be doing great work while keeping a vital momentum going. Work can be replicated easily. The key to doing great work is finding what makes an organization thrive and stand out.[158]

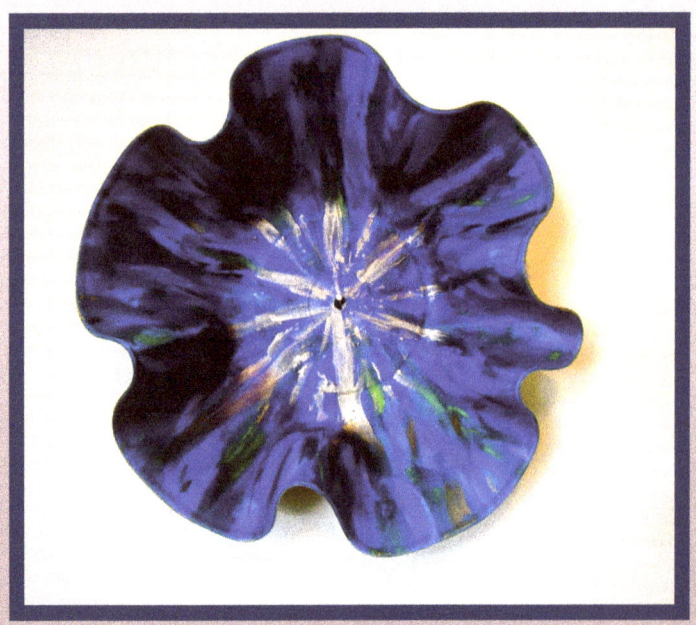

Courtesy of Rachel Brown

Today I will consider how I can stand out for the great work that I do. You are valuable to your company because ... Make a list of things in your journal that you do that contribute to the mission of your organization. Knowing your value is quite helpful when being evaluated for your performance.

MAY 28

Day 148

Being Intentional

Your life consists of choices. Each morning, you wake up to a day full of new opportunities and decisions. You pick your attitude and preferences. You do not have to allow the negative circumstances of your past to determine your future. You have options – don't continue the same patterns in your life that you have been struggling with for many years. Wake up every morning with a mindset open to new opportunities.[159]

Today I will evaluate my choices. Have I made wise decisions? If so, great. If not, then consider your openness to change. Journal about your life choices and the outcomes that have followed. Describe a time you were intentional about an attitude or a decision you made.

Courtesy of Carrie Shank

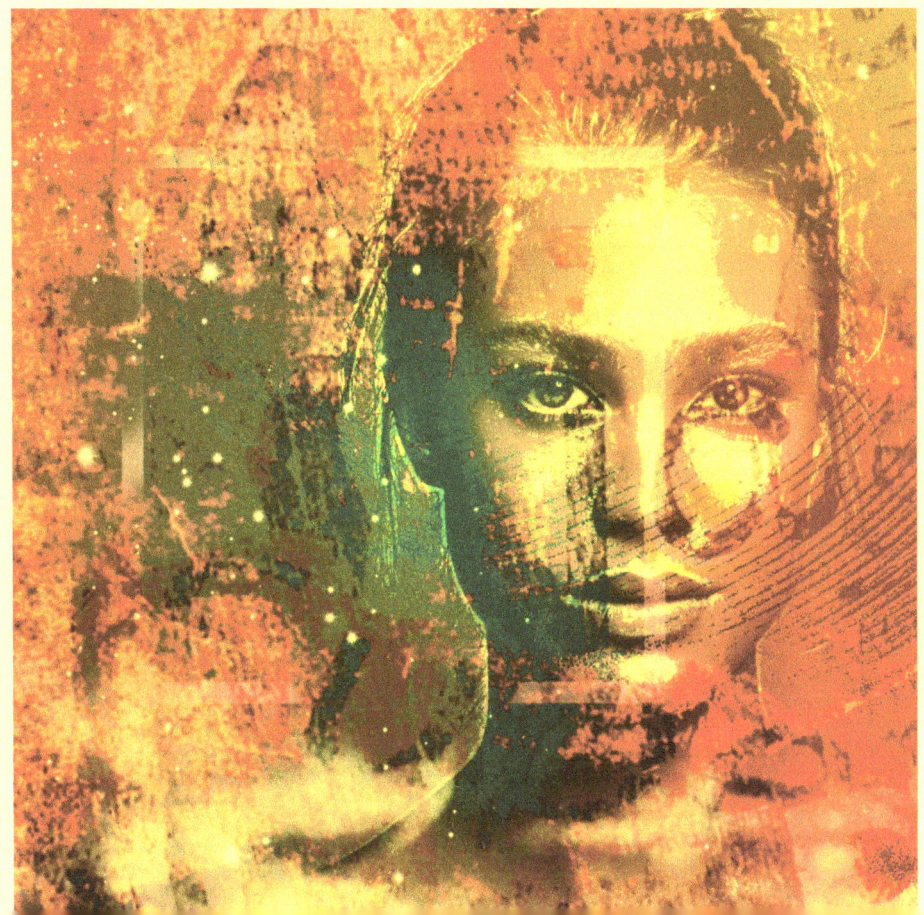

MAY 29

Day 149

My Ideas

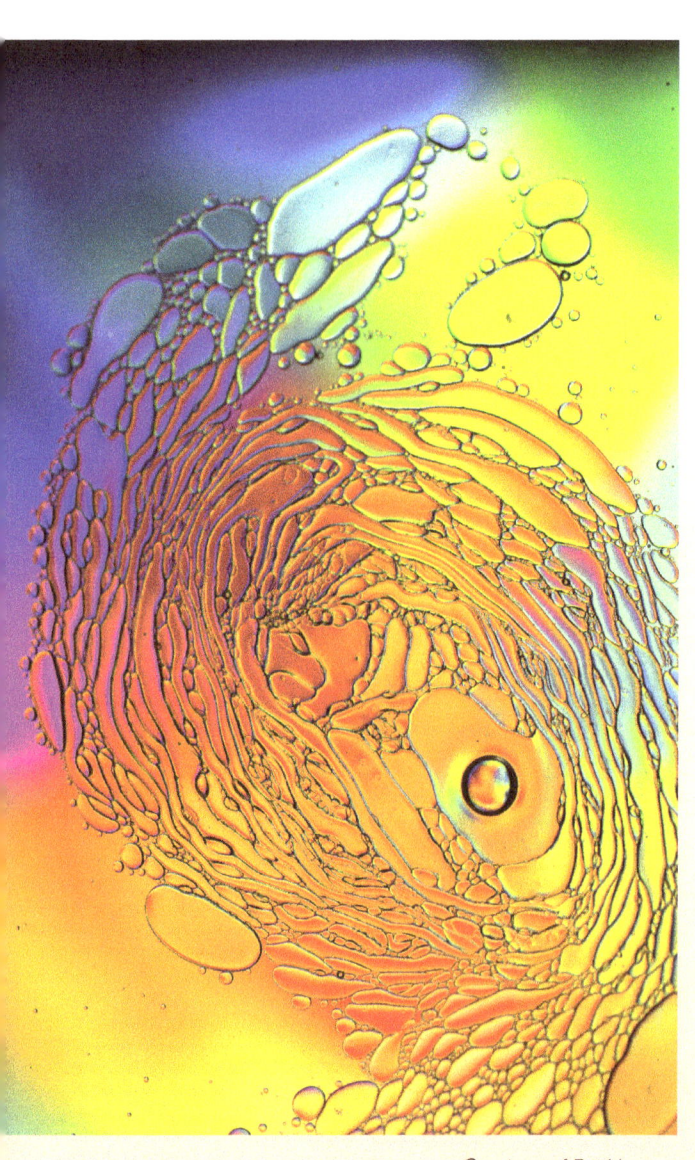

Courtesy of Patti Larson

When exercising your mind, no matter what focus, don't be fearful of expressing your thoughts. You just might stumble upon brilliant ideas. Educating yourself presents opportunities for discovering and allowing your mind to wander. Will your ideas belong to the past, what is still to come, or nothing at all? You'll probably reject most ideas that you have, which isn't a bad thing. When you continuously come up with new ideas, you should anticipate that most will pass by.[160]

Today I will consider my ideas. So much of what we do each day may be rote and uncreative. Let your mind wander in your free time. Try to relax and create in your mind; it relieves stress. What do you see? What brilliant ideas can you write about in your journal? Your ideas can turn into new opportunities. List three new bright ideas.

MAY 30

Day 150

Be Curious

Lacking motivation is not due to laziness or an absence of goals. Everyone can get lost sometimes - even those who some look up to, such as Hollywood stars, wealthy professionals, and the most talented athletes. People are motivated by their curiosity and how much faster or better they can be. Above all, be curious, and allow curiosity to drive you to goal attainment and success.[161]

Today I will reflect on my own curiosity. There is the old cliché that "curiosity killed the cat," but how often is this true? Without a certain amount of curiosity, motivation to excel at your goals would be narrow. When motivation is challenging, it nurtures your inner curiosity. Journal about a time when your curiosity helped you find the motivation to push you forward toward your goals. Do you consider yourself curious?

Courtesy of Ann Parker

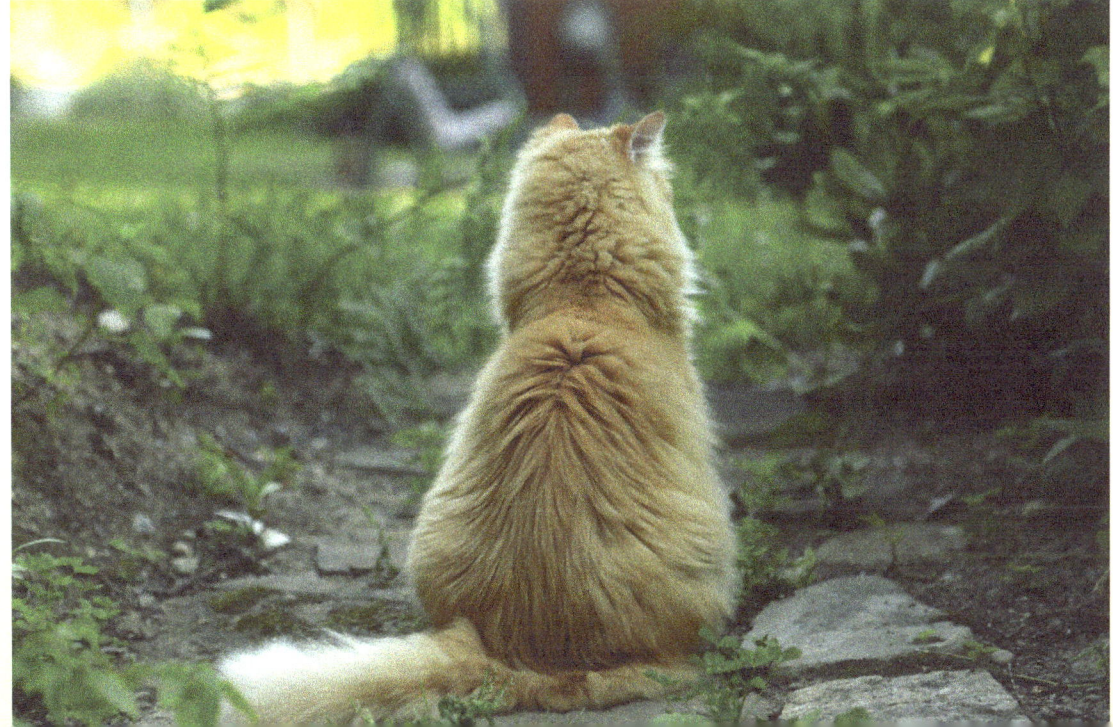

MAY 31

Day 151

My Full Potential

Rewarding careers will have their share of joys and disappointments, including bad days, weeks, and even months. Everyone faces setbacks and situations that are discouraging. Some people will abandon their goals and plans once they come across challenges. It is common for people to get lost and undermine their accomplishments, which is extra painful since it is self-induced. No one can stop you from reaching your full potential. The challenge you must face is recognizing your dreams, establishing what skills will get you there, and displaying leadership characteristics. Next, you must be courageous and occasionally reassess, adjust, and follow the course that truly represents who you are.[162]

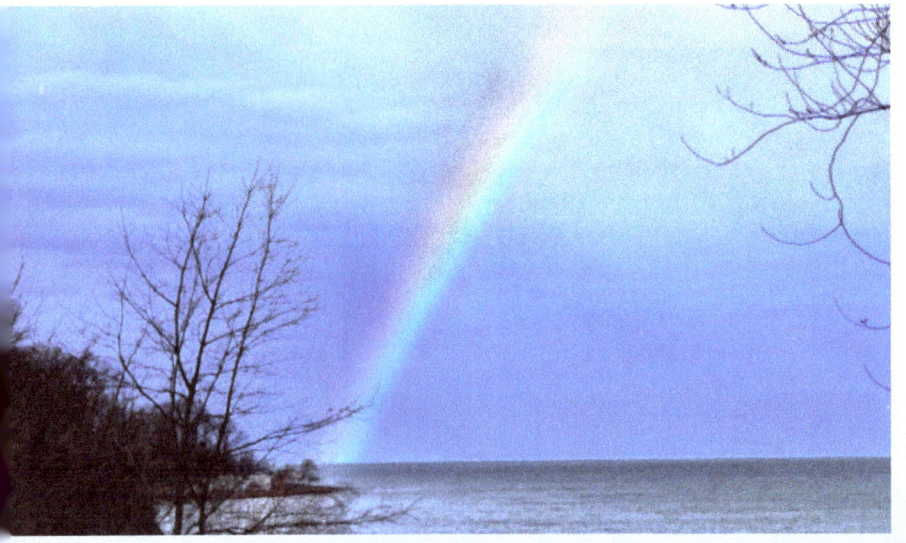

Courtesy of Spar Ki

Today I will consider whether I have reached my full potential or not. Awareness of your potential needs to be personal, not external. Staying right where you are in work and life is a comfortable thing. At some stages in life, the urge to reach further dissipates. Enjoying your now and where you are at home and work may be enough. But what if it isn't? Journal about how it might be time to adjust and make plans for developing yourself. What are some things you would like to enhance to reach your full potential that won't cause too much stress?

JUNE 1

Day 152

Being Thankful

What is on your list of blessings? You might be surprised at all the wonderful things you are grateful for. No need to include materialism, which is meaningless and shallow. What are the things you can focus on that are free, joyful, and offer humility? In your list, might you include your family, friends, body, mind, nature, faith, intellect, or pets? The list can be quite long.[163]

Today I will consider all that I am thankful for at home and work. Few of us take time to really be thankful for the little things we have like clean water, food, and shelter. Make a list in your journal at the start of your day. Maybe you're thankful for your dog or cat. Maybe you're grateful for your friends and family. Maybe you're thankful for your coworkers, your boss, your employees. Whatever and whoever it is, focus on the joy you feel and be specific. Telling someone you are thankful doesn't need to be stressful or too much work.

Courtesy of Jill Santi

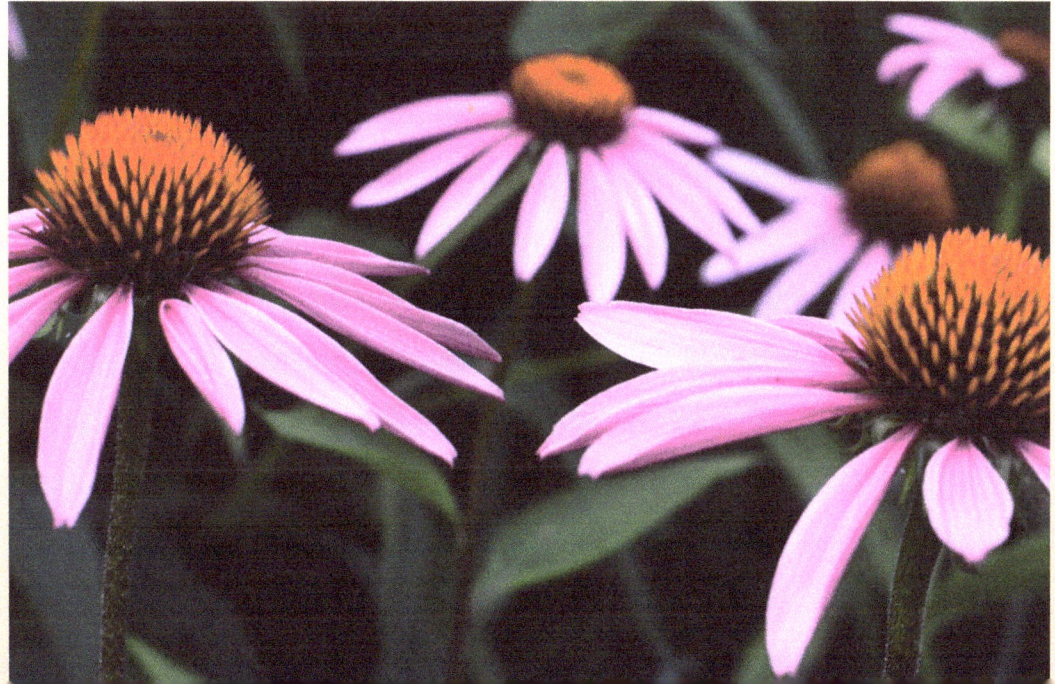

JUNE 2
Day 153

Expressing Concerns

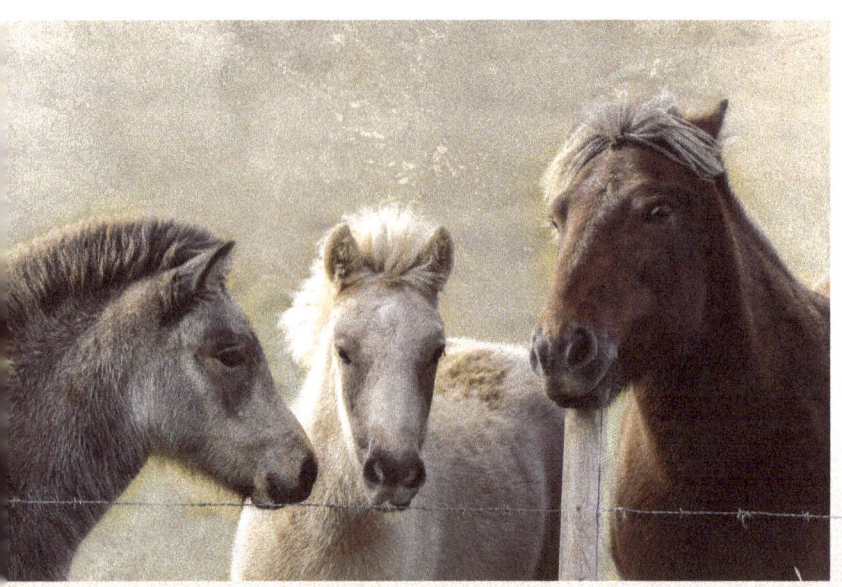

Courtesy of Patti Larson

Today I will reflect on a conversation I have wanted to have with someone. Maybe it's a conversation about uncomfortable things you don't want to deal with. Maybe it's an issue that has been ignored in the past. Being able to communicate without getting frustrated or angry is a measure of being emotionally aware. Expressing your messages of concern requires planning. When pointed conversations are unplanned, it can create a stressful situation. Decide which difficult conversation is pressing you today, and in your journal, plan key points you want to address.

Problems range from workflow inabilities to conflicts with personalities. Employees usually are privy to and observe drama and system failures, yet they may feel unable to discuss certain concerns with management or executives who can intervene. While being reluctant to cause an upset is understandable, employees should know that many leaders within organizations respect hearing about concerns, even from new hires. Discussing process errors, drama, and personal accommodations may not always be simple, but planning those types of conversations is wise. [164]

JUNE 3

Day 154

Challenges Into Opportunities

With any crisis, you tend to see the emergence of talented, unidentified leaders. Those with the correct talent and skill set will confront challenges in a crisis, even if they are not recognized as top performers. This creates a dynamic that encourages the entire staff to improve camaraderie and work together efficiently.[165]

Today I will think about turning my challenges into opportunities. Journal about your top three challenges. Which one is the priority? Which can you overcome single-handedly? Which challenges do you need help with, and which can you rise to meet and tackle today? When there are too many challenges, how does that impact camaraderie and efficiency?

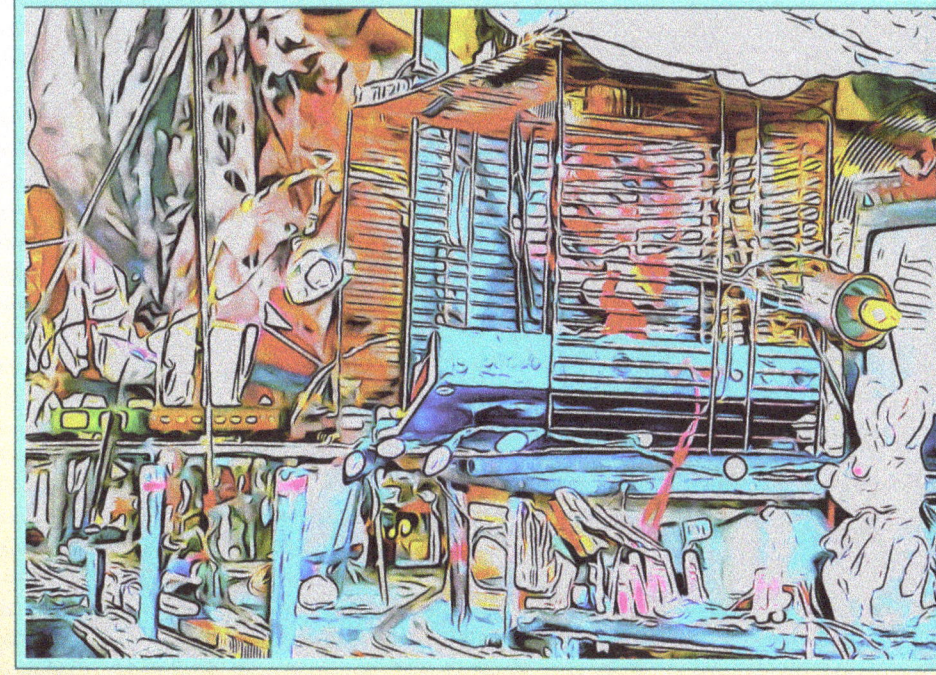

Courtesy of Robert John Holland

JUNE 4
Day 155

Networking

The word "networking" gives many a feeling of dread. However, a lot of research has suggested that networking in a positive manner affects success. Having robust and diverse social and professional networks will lead to better jobs, open us to new ideas and profitable arenas, and even help us get better pay. While traditional network approaches of going to events and asking for advice can be productive, it is getting tougher to use this approach to build stronger and successful relationships. Those who are influential are busy and aren't inclined to meet people lower on the power structure. Many are overloaded with requests and have assistants securing their schedules.[166]

Today I will consider the networking expectations placed on me and how that may create some stress. For introverts, the last thing they want to do is network with other people. Introverts typically like working alone with the projects that interest them. What are your thoughts on networking? Journal about whether you consider yourself to be more of an introvert or extrovert. If you are an introvert, how can you build a strong, successful network? Extroverts are quite skilled at networking and do so effortlessly. Introverts need to work at improving their relationship skills.

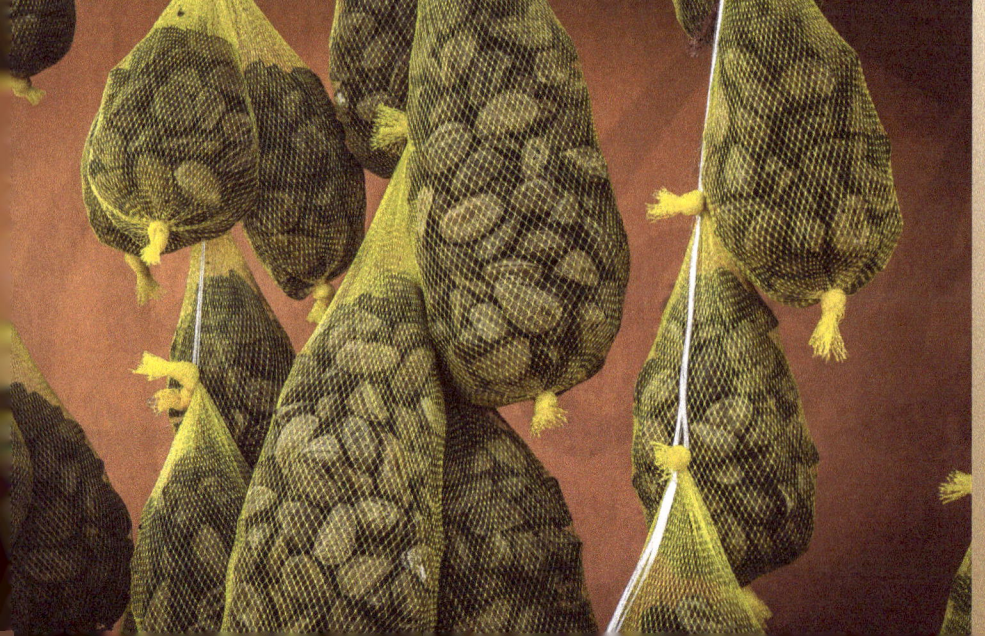

Courtesy of Mara Rubin

JUNE 5

Day 156

Making Peace

Creating peace within the world requires a change of consciousness to becoming a peacemaker yourself. Anyone can do it. Reach within and commit to peaceful thoughts, speeches, actions, and healthy relationships with others.[167]

Today and each day, I will seek peace. Being peaceful will hopefully make the world reciprocate peace. In a world where there may be contentious issues that create war, it takes conscious effort to make peace, have peace, and keep peace. What can you do to show others you are a loving or non-violent person? Do calm feelings help you sustain healthy relationships? Journal about your thoughts on peace and capturing it, now.

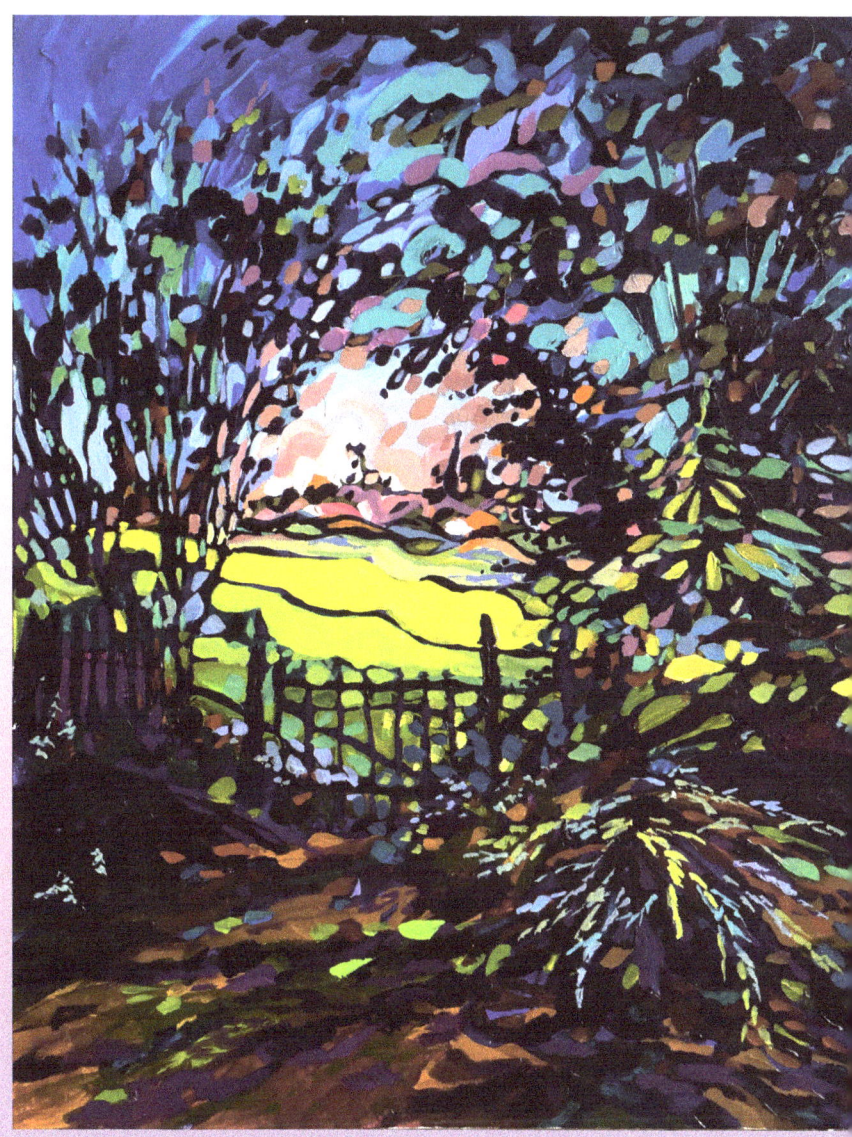

Courtesy of Judy Hodge

JUNE 6

Day 157

Frustration

When you are blocked from a goal, you may feel frustrated. Frustration may feel destructive as an emotion but often becomes creative fuel. When frustrated, we question the status quo, reject how things have been done, and discover improved and new methods. Dissatisfaction promotes creativity if people are committed to teamwork and obtain the support needed for pursuing their ideas.[168]

Today I will consider if I am being blocked from a goal. Is a person(s), place, or other barrier stopping you from achieving your desired result or moving forward in your career goals? Is there something you are doing to block yourself? Feeling frustrated is annoying and not a good thing to dwell on. At some point, the frustration will hit a turning point or boiling point. Frustration is stressful, and can create emotional exhaustion and perhaps burnout if not countered with healthy self-care. Journal about a time you felt frustrated and what you did to overcome it.

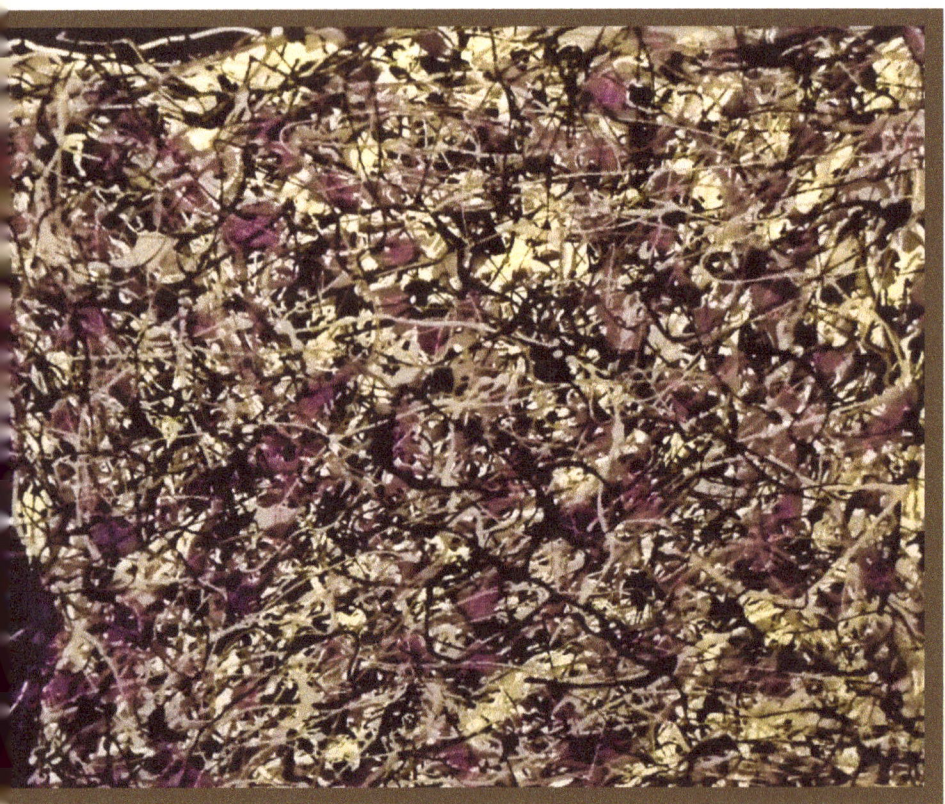

Courtesy of Aryn Grayson

JUNE 7
Day 158

Venting

Even though venting can feel good at times, it can feel a bit unprofessional as well. Within high-stress and high-stake professions, blowing off steam often makes sense and can be a positive thing; however, it may also carry negative energy. Ultimately, risks tend to exceed the benefits. There are usually more suitable means of pursuing support.[169]

Today I will consider that venting can be very tempting to do but it may not be the most positive thing for me in the long run, especially at work. Yes, talking about concerns and bringing them forward professionally is essential for creating new ways of improving circumstances. However, be careful about how you "vent" to others and how you may be perceived. Journal about a time at work when you vented. Did it have a positive, negative, or absent result? When venting causes a negative result, it can often increase stress and tension within the workplace.

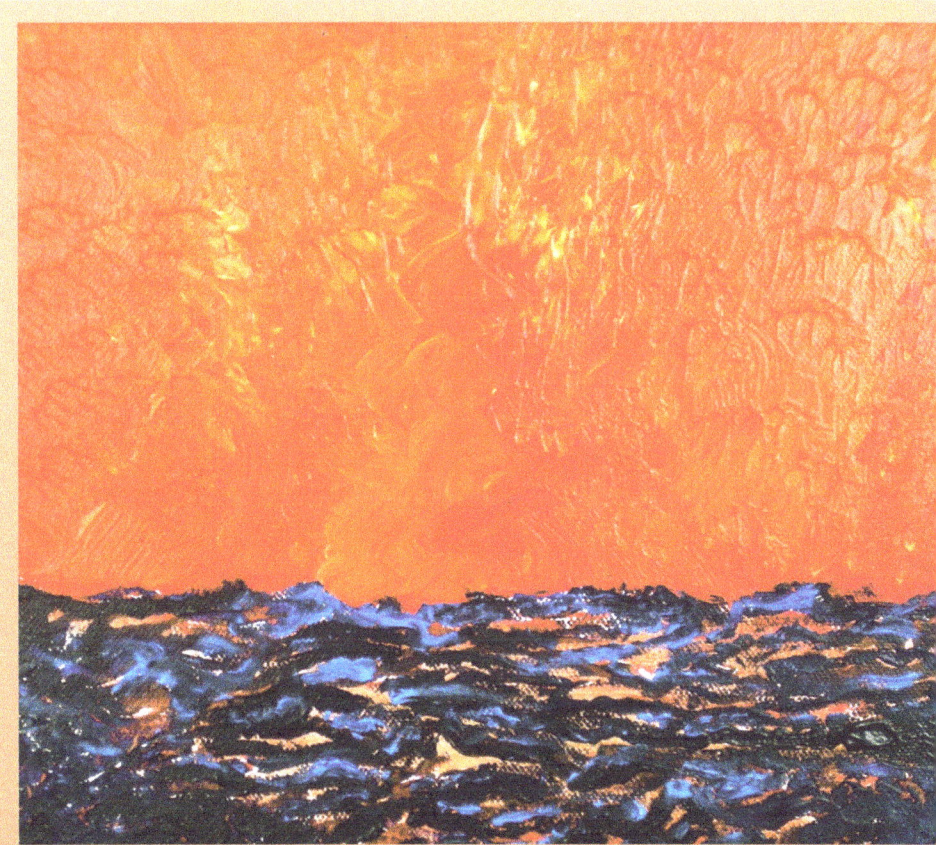

Courtesy of Peter Sterling Turner

JUNE 8

Day 159

Nothing Ventured, Nothing Gained

"The first known reference to this quote is in 'The Reeve's Tale' (c.1476), one of the stories in Geoffrey Chaucer's The Canterbury Tales."[170] Without taking any risks, a person may be unable to achieve anything throughout life. Subsequently, only those with the courage to act and achieve something in their lives, even when the future is not guaranteed, will become successful.[171]

Today I will consider whether I am the type of person to take risks without knowing the outcome. If you don't take risks, do you gain security, peace of mind, or perhaps monotony? Would you feel dissatisfaction, frustration, or stress with your predicament if you don't take a risk? Maybe a new venture is in order, and maybe not. What project or endeavor can you create? Do you want to create a new venture? Write about your answers in your journal.

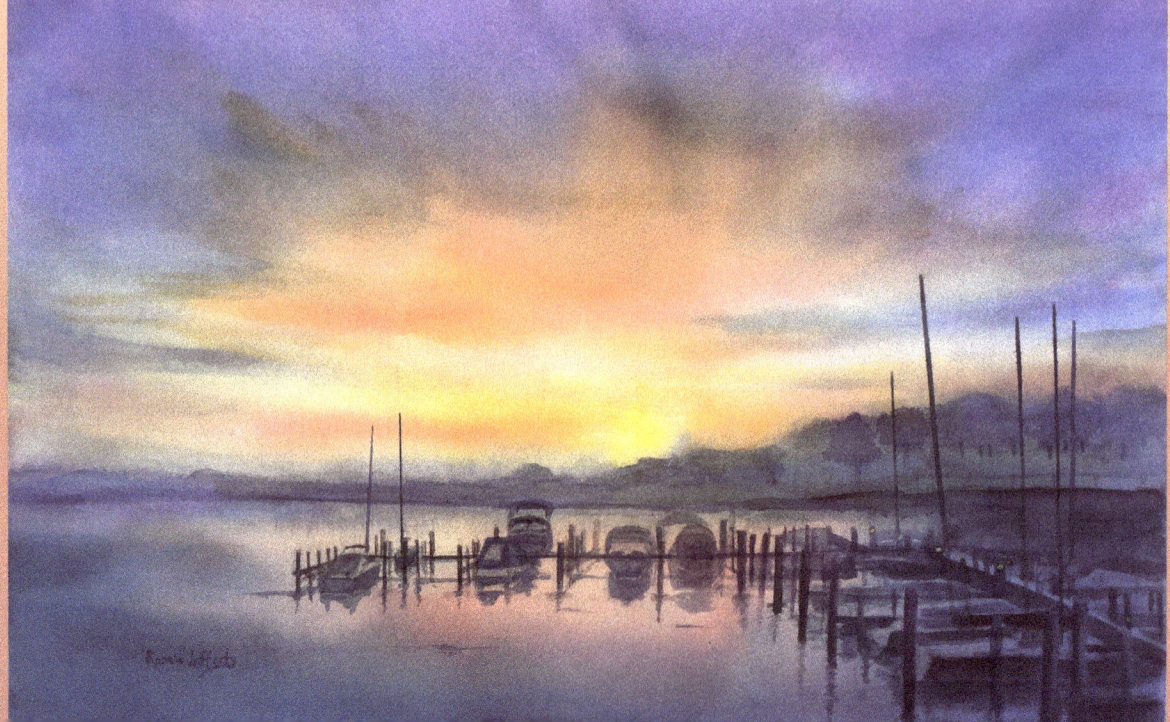

Courtesy of Ronnie Lafferty

JUNE 9

Day 160

Being Prepared

Being prepared guarantees readiness for when a disaster may strike. It is universally vital to be prepared for anything. Emergencies can strike anywhere, including at home or work. Everyone must be sure to plan for when unexpected situations occur. You must be prepared for anything to happen all 365 days of the year. Take charge and control of a situation as much as you can by being prepared.[172]

Today I will think about whether I am prepared for any emergency at home or work. Do you have a specific plan for the unexpected in place? What if there were a flood, tornado, fire, pandemic, or any other unthinkable disaster? When you have a plan in place, there is less stress because everyone knows what to do, including you. If you don't have emergency plans, today is a good day to start making them. Journal about plans you can make to prepare for any future emergency.

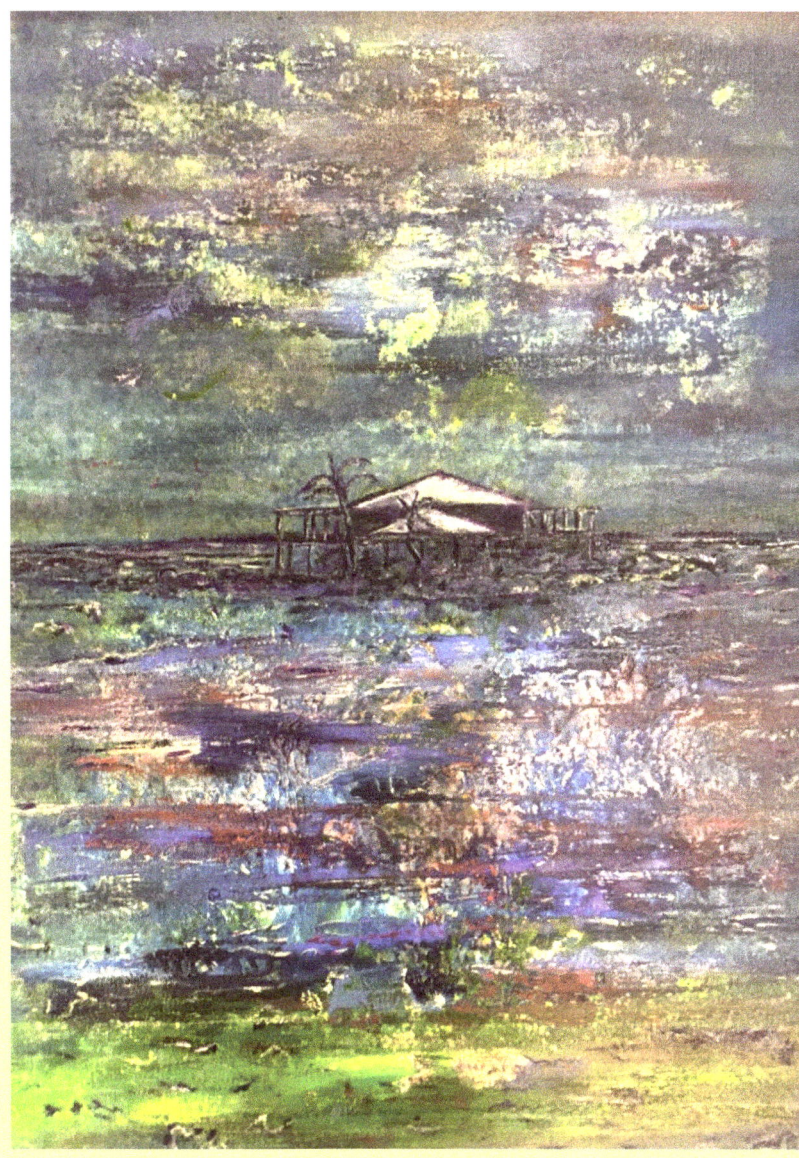

Courtesy of Peter Sterling Turner

JUNE 10
Day 161

Develop Your Own Career Strategy

Making decisions related to your career doesn't just happen one time. We make life-long progressive steps in a developmental process. On average, workers change careers three times and jobs seven times throughout their life. Companies that are successful make strategic plans providing aspirational long-term visions. They have specific goals and objectives, which incrementally bring them toward realizing their vision. This process can parallel the development of your own successful career management strategy.[173]

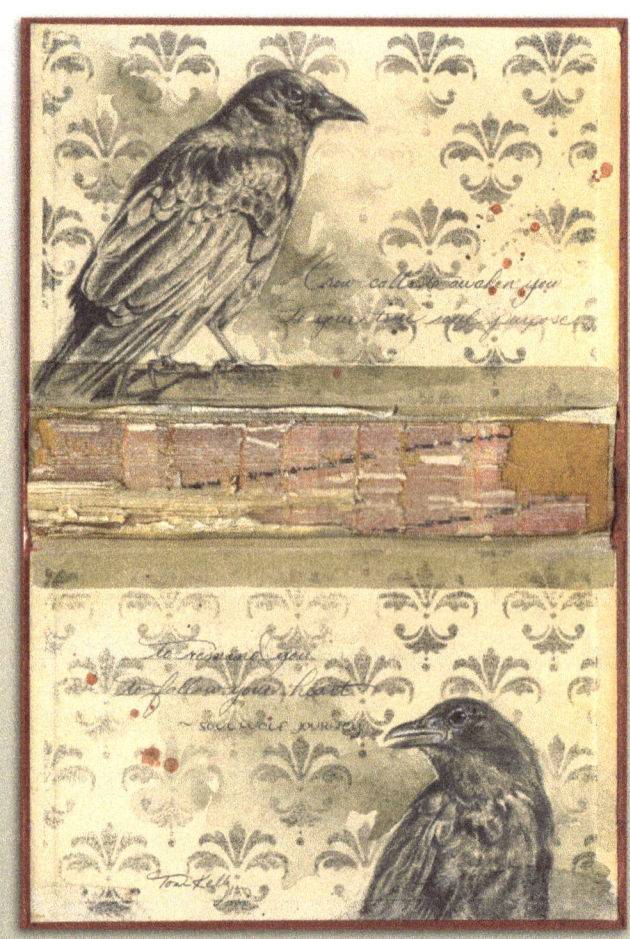

Courtesy of Toni Kelly

Today I will consider if I am content where I am at with my career. Do you know where you want to be in one, two, or five years from now? What plans can you make for yourself developing your own career strategy? How can you alleviate some of your stress by having a plan for your future? Journal about your short and long term goals, now.

Day 162 — JUNE 11

Your Brand

Many people don't want to have a personal brand. They would rather allow their work to speak for itself. Many argue that after working 20 plus years, why should it be required to self-promote now, especially if there is no interest? The downside is that even if you say, "I don't want to have a personal brand," you don't get much of a say in that nowadays. When heading outside on a bright, sunny day, your body automatically casts your shadow. Personal branding happens and works in much the same way.[174]

Today I will consider upgrading my personal brand. Think of it as a public identity that leaves a first and lasting impression on the people you meet and work with. Pressure to develop your own personal brand can be stressful if it isn't something that you understand or want. Journal about a time you may have felt the pressure of dealing with personal branding. Do you feel or think your work should speak for itself? Read an article on personal branding, then make a simple plan for creating your brand today.

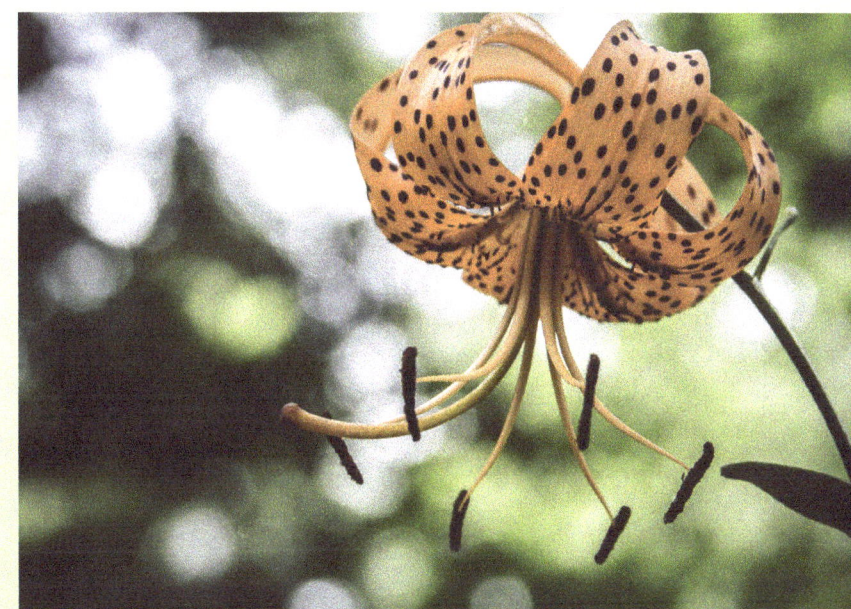

Courtesy of Mara Rubin

JUNE 12
Day 163

Feel Good

Some things you can do to feel good are:
- Monitor your stress level
- Enjoy your own self
- Increase your self-esteem
- Enjoy simple activities
- Commit to a healthy lifestyle
- Exercise
- Choose healthy foods
- Talk and share
- Get enough rest
- Build your grit[175]

Today I will feel good. Do the best you can to let go of all the stresses in your life. If you can, take a walk outside. De-stress from exhaustion at work. You deserve to feel good every day, but do you? If not, what things can you do to feel better? Write your answers in your journal about "feeling good."

Courtesy of Nancy Nixon Ensign

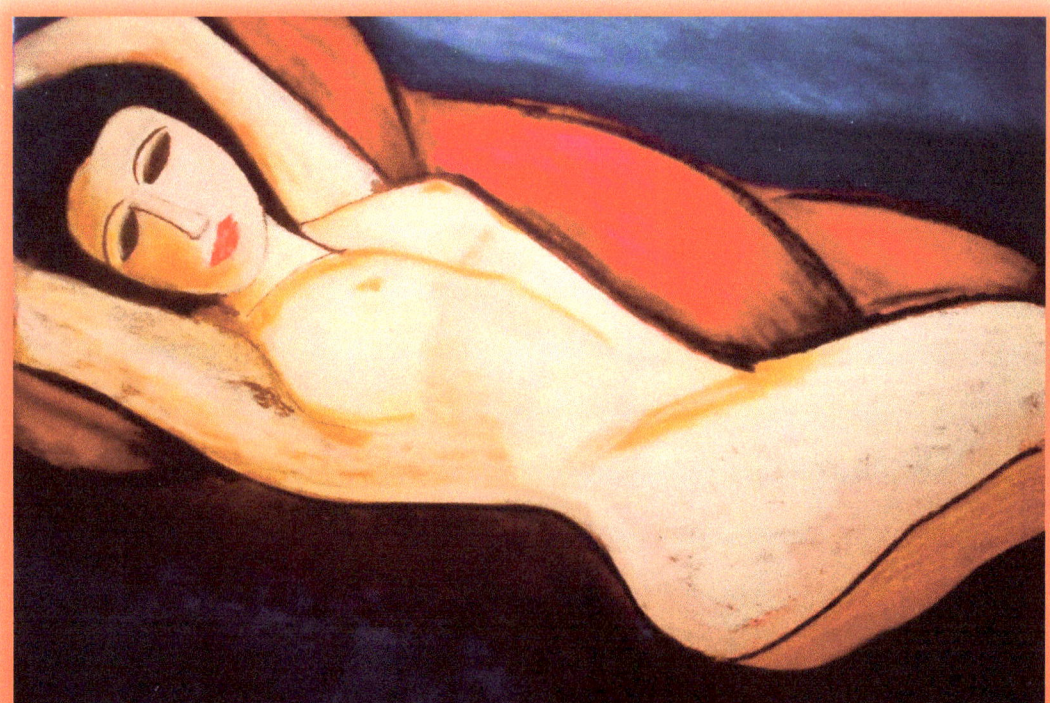

JUNE 13

Day 164

Social Awareness

Being socially aware allows people to share their perspectives while having the ability to empathize with diverse cultural differences. Understanding other backgrounds, behavioral norms, and ethics is helpful. Recognizing different types of family dynamics, schools, and community resources builds a supportive social awareness. Awareness of other perspectives is also a critical element of proper classroom etiquette, which supports an environment for learning. Social awareness is widely accepted as a necessary factor for workplace success.[176]

Today I will consider whether I am a socially aware individual. Do you think about others in the room and how they perceive you? Do you exhibit empathy in a world where it is nearly nonexistent? Look around and see what others are going through. It isn't always all about you. While it is important to maintain your boundaries and prioritize yourself to some degree, you can also think about and care for others. Journal about a time you thought of someone other than yourself and were able to show empathy for their situation. What did you do to show you care? What was their reaction?

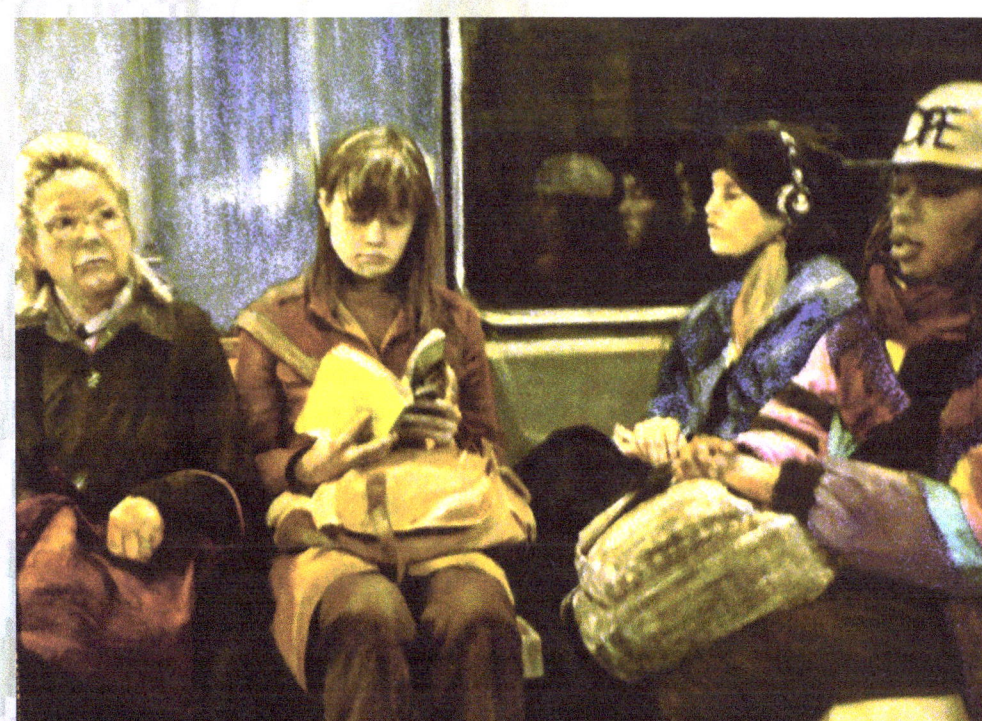

Courtesy of Susan MacKay

Day 165

JUNE 14

Tone, Volume, and Cadence

Creating sound is accomplished by applying the voice while using words to render speech. When people listen to you, they connect your voice as a piece of what you ascribe to and your identity. You can use your voice to whisper, mutter, or shout. You can use your voice to suggest, demand, and roar. You can announce, state, assert, affirm, and declare. You'll be judged by the credibility and sincerity people hear in your voice.[177]

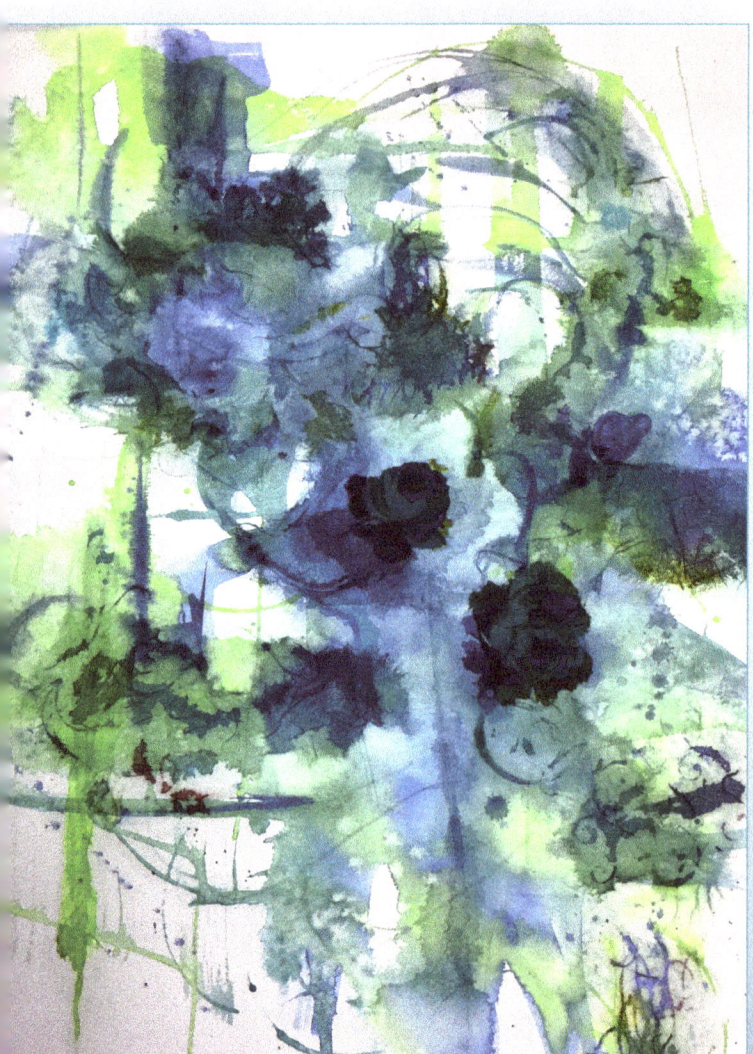

Today I will think about my voice and how I use it for good. Adjust your tone, volume, and cadence to be appropriate. You can influence others to either remain calm or panic during stressful situations, all by using your voice. Being assertive begins with your voice. The quality of your pitch, timbre, rhythm, tempo, and emotional expression also capture the listener's attention and support. Journal about a recent time you demonstrated believability and earnestness, all by using your voice.

Courtesy of Ronnie Lafferty

JUNE 15

Day 166

Legitimate Concerns

Sometimes you don't agree with things on the job, and while some do not like to complain, it may be inevitable. You might need to give negative feedback on legitimate concerns, which may be difficult for someone to hear. It's best to have optimal timing when voicing your concerns. Try to be specific, objective, and let go of emotional attachment. Always have some solutions in mind and try to focus on what is positive. Remember to leave the decision making to your boss and get some support if you need it.[178]

Today I will consider my legitimate concerns and take the necessary steps to address them. You can't go on indefinitely feeling silenced about things that may be occurring that are a cause for apprehension. That is both stressful and exhausting. Don't be afraid to speak up. Journal about a time you had to address your legitimate concerns and the outcome.

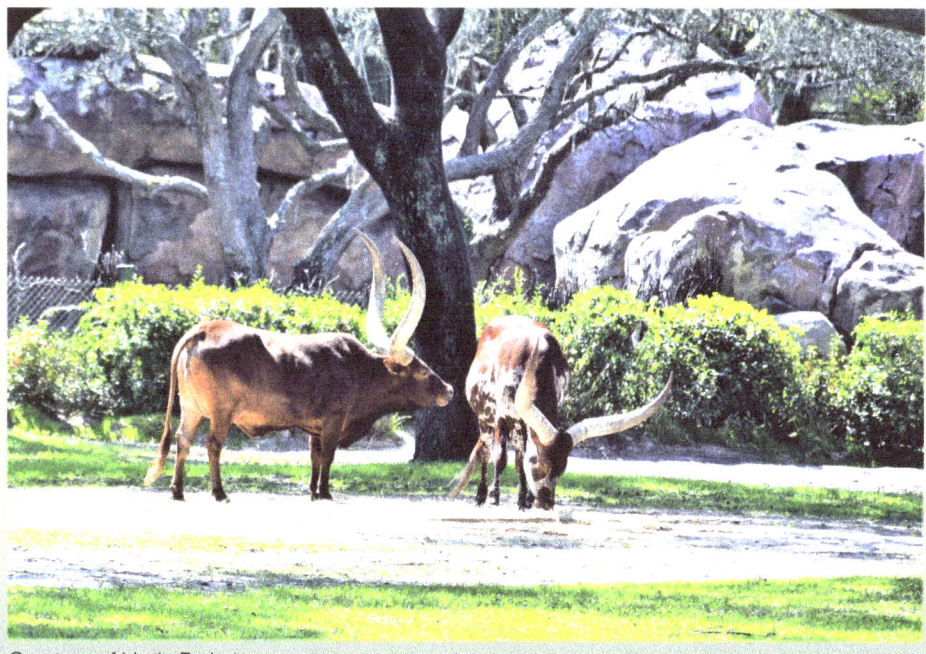

Courtesy of Linda Probst

JUNE 16
Day 167

Addictions

Burnout is intense, and it can threaten your health as well as your career and relationship. It can often drag on for years. People keep pushing through their feelings of intense physical, emotional, and mental exhaustion. It is relatively easy to recognize how burnout is often an underlying cause of addiction.[179]

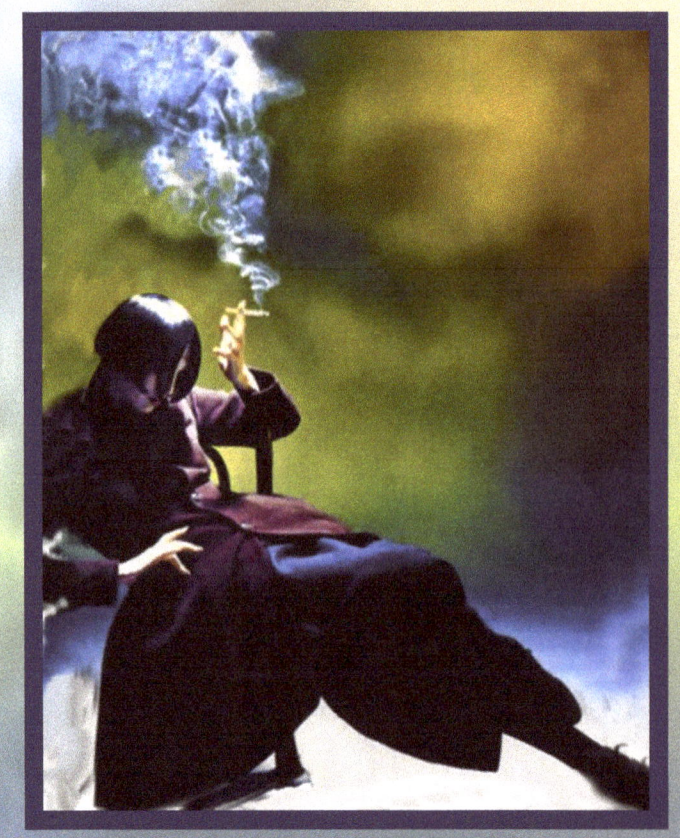

Courtesy of Susan MacKay

Today I will consider addictions. Do you use substances? Drugs and alcohol are problematic. Burnout may be an underlying reason for addiction. You can take the first step to recovery if you allow yourself to ask for help by calling the Substance Abuse and Mental Health Services Administration (SAMHSA)'s National Helpline – 1-800-662-HELP (4357). In your journal, write about someone you know (or maybe yourself) that suffered or is suffering from an addiction. Is it affecting physical, emotional, and mental wellbeing?

JUNE 17
Day 168

Types of Burnout

There are different types of burnout. Overload burnout describes people that work frantically, searching for success. Often, they risk their own health and priorities in their personal life. They pursue ambition and complain in order to cope. Under-challenge burnout describes a lack of opportunities to learn, feeling unappreciated, and being bored. These people no longer find enjoyment or passion in their job and will distance themselves from their work. They are indifferent, cynical, avoid responsibility, and are disengaged. Neglect burnout occurs when people feel helpless at work. Demands in the workplace make them feel incompetent and not able to stay focused. These workers may often be unmotivated and passive.[180]

Today I will consider which type of burnout I may be experiencing. Are you overloaded, under-challenged, or feeling helpless with your job demands? Are you experiencing more than one type of burnout? Where and when did your burnout originate? In your journal, describe what you have been doing to reduce feelings of burnout. Don't neglect your self-care.

Courtesy of Ann Parker

JUNE 18

Day 169

Being Truthful, Not Hurtful

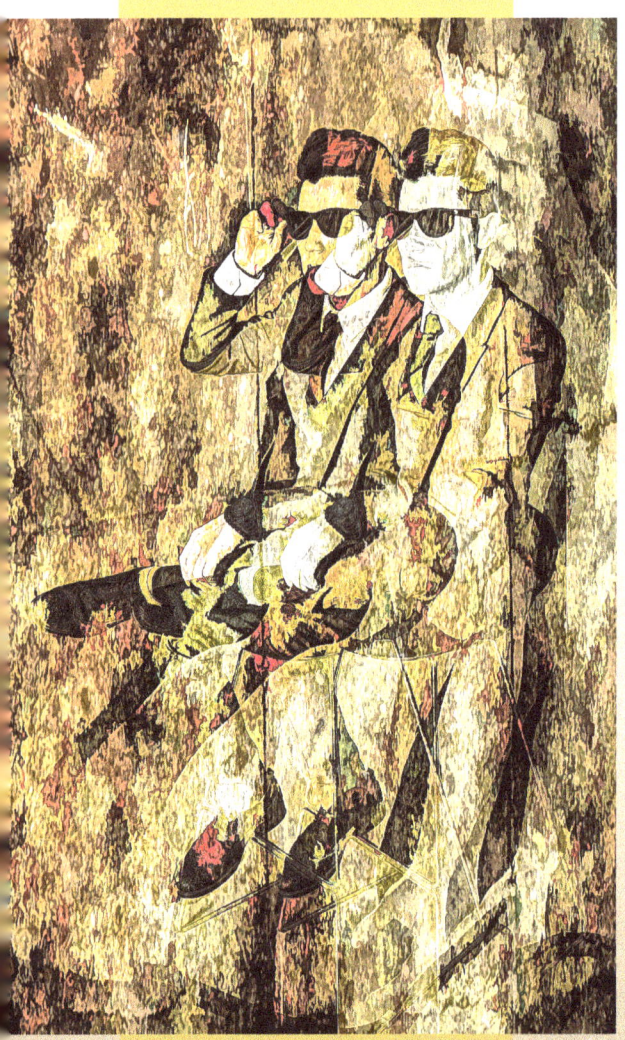

Courtesy of Carrie Shank

Honesty is often the best policy. Only your best friends can truly be honest with you most times. It is a safe assumption that only those who genuinely care for you the most have the courage to bring you the actual truth, even when it can be hurtful. However, many other people make it a point to purposely be mean and hurt you for the sake of "honesty," which is not the same. There is a thin, distinct line between the two scenarios.[181]

Today I will consider being truthful, not hurtful. I will remember to give constructive criticism without being perceived as mean or negative. Sometimes people can be hurtful, though, which does cause tension. Journal about a time you were truthful without being hurtful recently. What was the situation? Honesty is the best policy, except when it is purposefully mean.

JUNE 19

Day 170

Belonging

There are studies that have shown a sense of belonging felt in the workplace can lead to much more than positive vibes and friendships. A sense of belonging allows workers to feel comfortable about their authentic self and not fear negative treatment or retribution. Belonging has a crucial impact on retention and performance. Inclusion and diversity are still important factors; however, we must realize that belonging is also a variable in the equation. It is a critical piece that leads to employee engagement as well as their psychological safety. A supportive environment may also trigger alternate responses within the brain, which leads to better ways of problem-solving.[182]

Today I will consider whether I feel belonging in my workplace. When you feel as if you belong, this leads to a sense of safety, authenticity, engagement, and loyalty to your work and team. Write about your thoughts regarding "belonging" both at work and home in your journal.

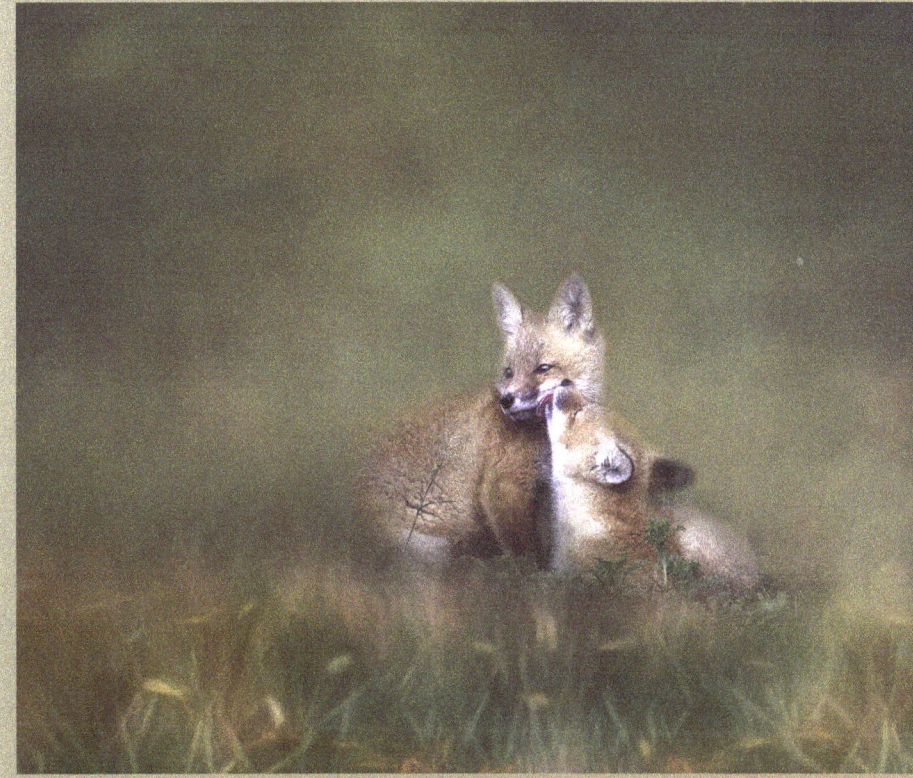

Courtesy of Patti Larson

JUNE 20
Day 171

Sticking With It

Experience can teach you certain things. The first is to pay attention to your gut feelings, even if something looks good on paper. The second is that you may be better off sticking to things you know. Third, sometimes better investments are those you do not make.[183]

Today I will think about "sticking with it." What does that mean? Sometimes, it's best to stick with what you know. Maybe it makes the most sense. Maybe not. Do you give up too early in the struggle with new projects? Journal and reflect on something you are sticking with that may cause either distress or joy.

Courtesy of Ann Parker

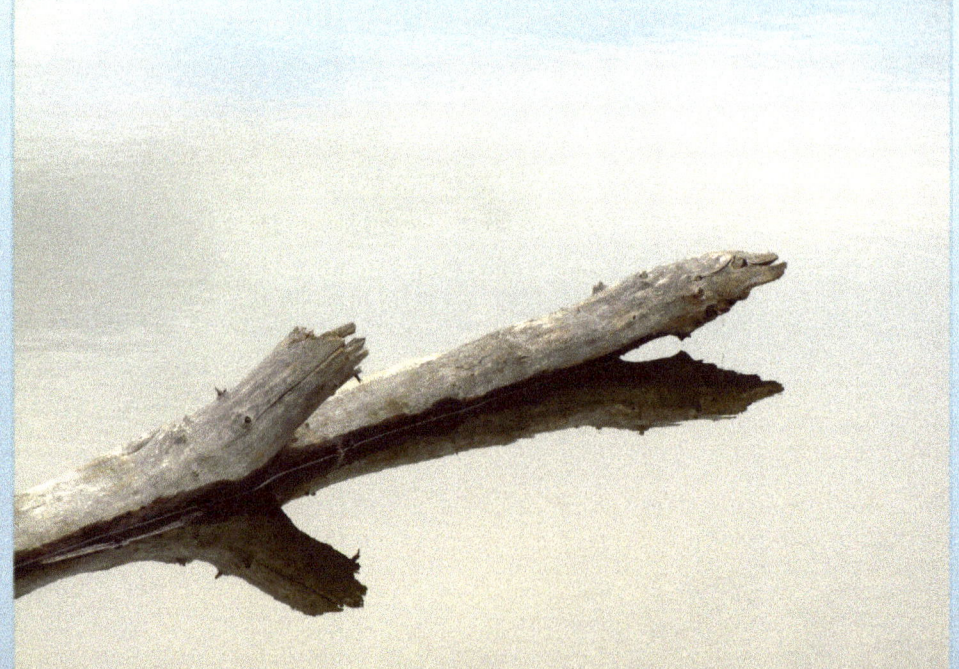

JUNE 21

Day 172

Being Denied Opportunities

Do you feel that you aren't learning, being challenged, or acquiring new skill sets? Does the boss want to maintain your position exactly where it is - right on the lower rung of the ladder? Is there a way to climb the ladder if someone is intentionally holding you back? Are you being denied opportunities?[184]

Today I will consider whether it is someone else or myself that is holding me back from growth. If it is your "boss," then it's time to have a professional conversation and understand why you are getting passed over, and it could be stressful. Maybe it's time to put a new action into place if you want to climb the ladder. Journal about what you think are your top three stumbling blocks to breaking the glass ceiling.

Courtesy of Mara Rubin

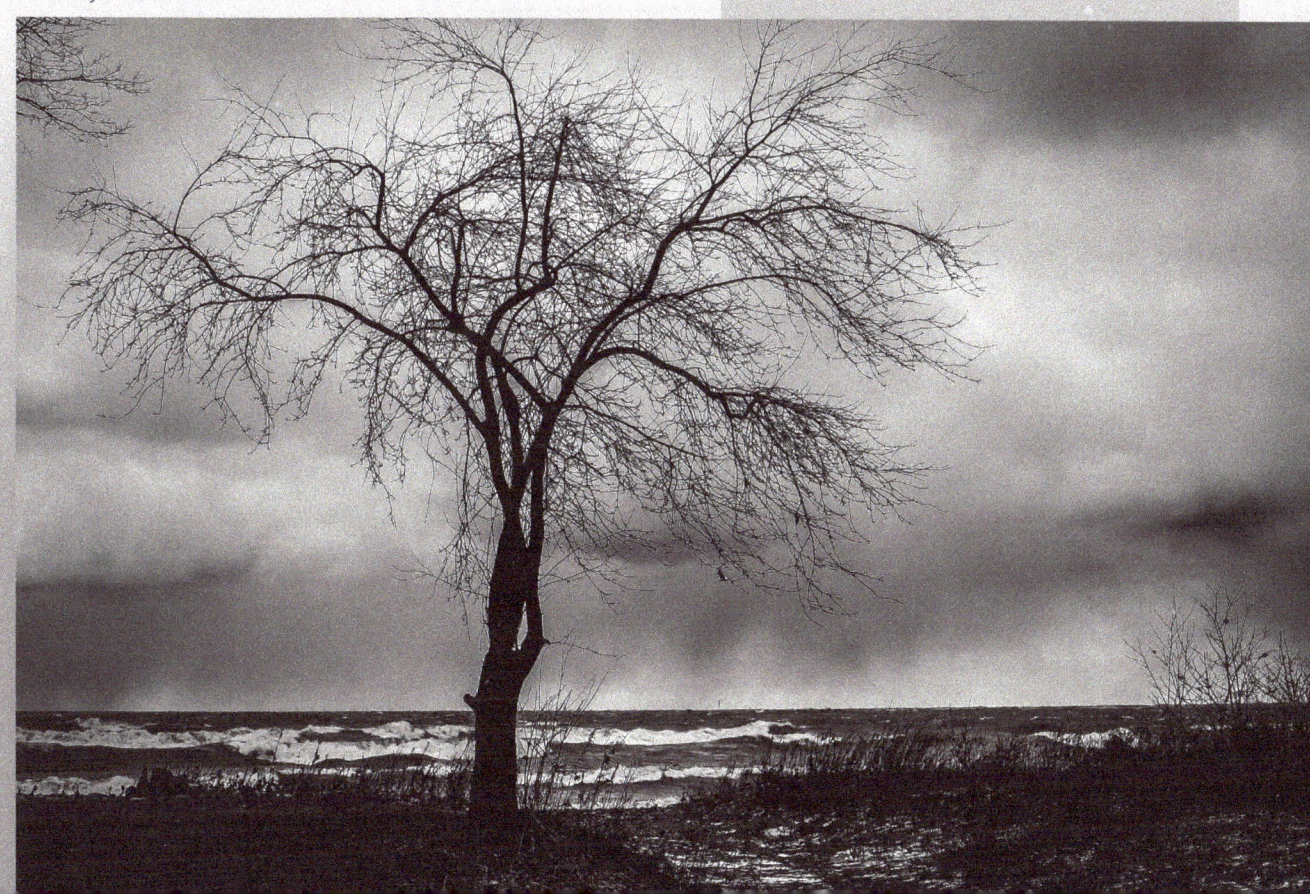

JUNE 22

Day 173

My Sleep Pattern

The exact definition of burnout is unclear. Burnout is not classified as a disease. There are no diagnostic standardized criteria for defining it. Authors may propose that burnout is less of a medical condition, and more of a circumstance linked between an employee and management expectations in the workplace. These mismatched beliefs are best approached through management techniques rather than medical treatment. Sleep problems, fatigue, cognitive impairment, and mood disorders appear to be the most frequent burnout symptoms.[185]

Today I will assess my sleep pattern. How did I sleep last night? What about this past week, month, or year? Journal about how you would rate the quality of your sleep. Is it poor, fair, good, or great? Know that having a poor sleep pattern is a symptom that could lead to burnout. Try to fix your sleep pattern by resting,

Courtesy of Nixon Ensign

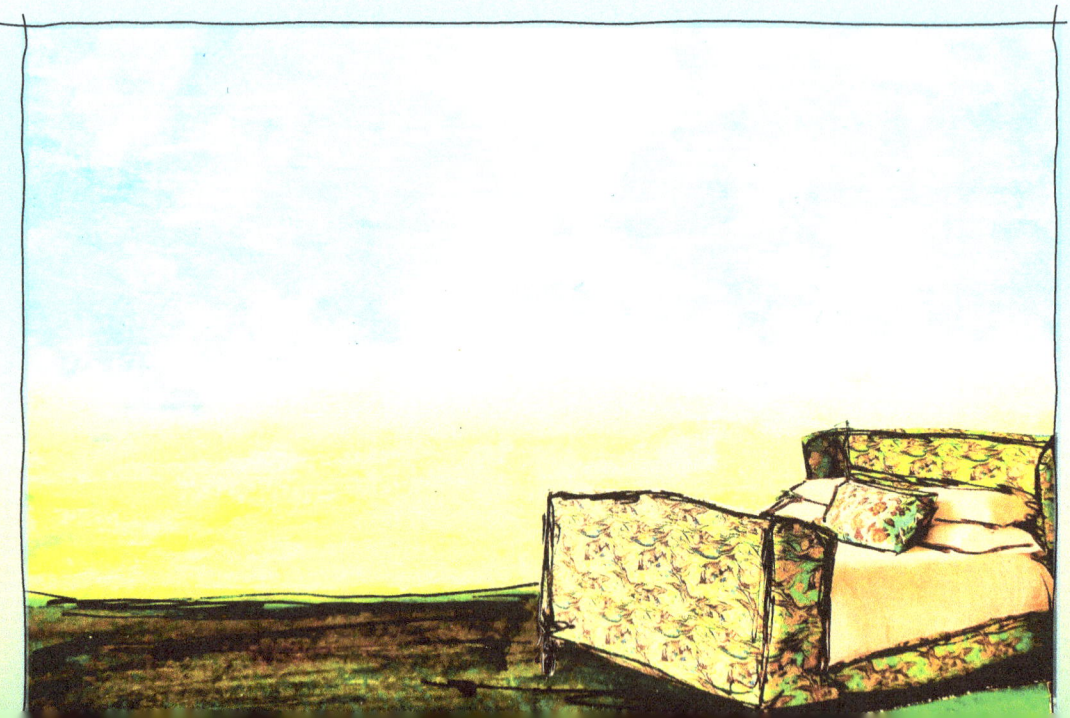

JUNE 23

Day 174

Taking Risks

Often, it can make sense to take risks when it involves your career. Taking risks just for the sake of it can be foolish, but there are many scenarios where safe choices limit your potential. If you take a risk and don't succeed, getting another job is a possibility. It might seem frightening, but if it's well thought out, the risk will often end up working out in your favor.[186]

Today I will think about the last time I took a risk in my career. Was it asking for or taking a promotion, finding a new level of responsibility in the same organization, or moving into a completely different job with another company? Having the courage to take on a new job or a new role is not easy for everyone. Some people are too stressed out about the idea of taking risks because of what they might lose along with added responsibilities at work or home. Calculating your risks is always the best option. Journal about the last time you took a risk and how it worked out for you. Was the risk worth taking? How did the outcome end up?

Courtesy of Linda Probst

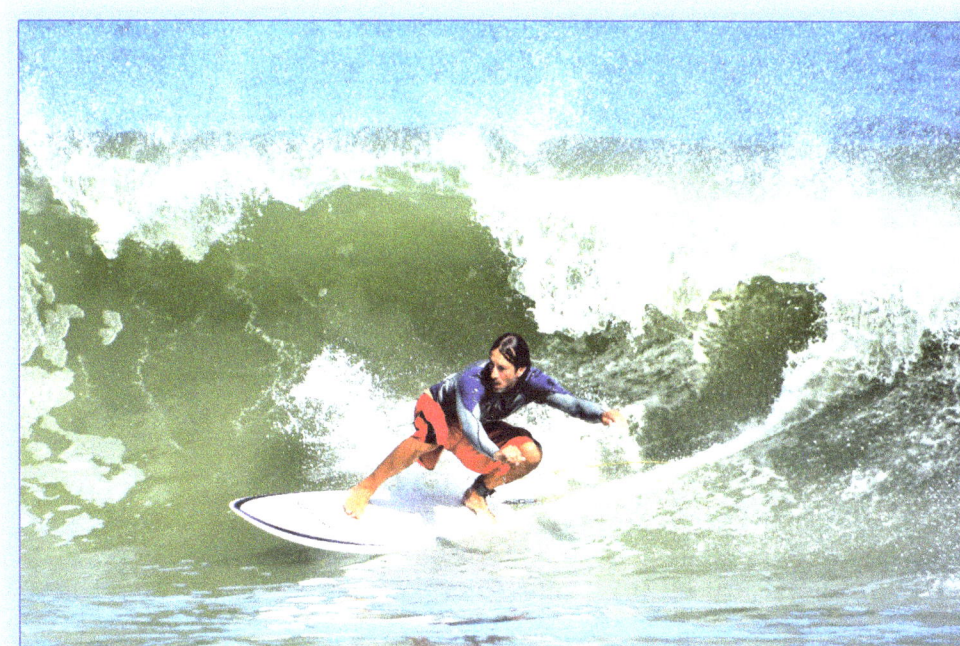

JUNE 24

Day 175

Unneccessary Drama

Drama within the workplace creates a tense environment. From office cliques to rumor mills, most of us have experienced this uncomfortable situation.[187]

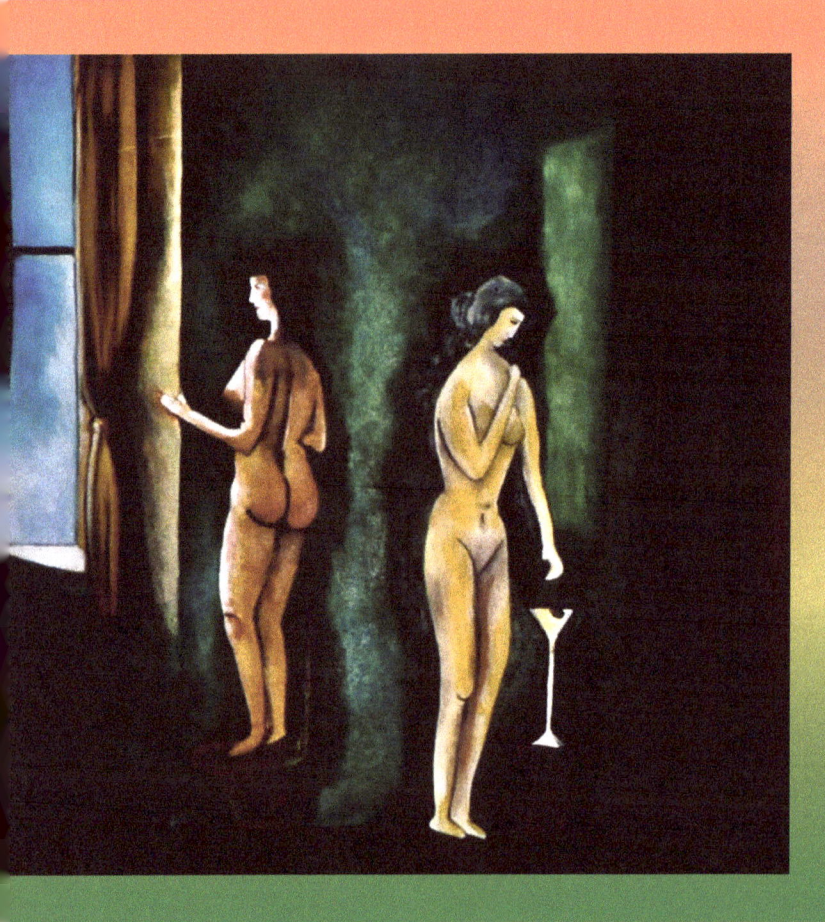

Courtesy of Nancy Nixon Ensign

Today I will consider whether I am taking part in unnecessary drama at work. Unnecessary drama is counterproductive and can be quite draining and stressful. Tell yourself that you won't engage in dramatic behaviors and focus on the work at hand to make the workplace better. Unnecessary drama can cause employees to separate instead of working together. Reflect on and journal about whether you bring unnecessary drama to work, or if others do, and how to remove it.

JUNE 25

Day 176

Being Humble

Humility tends to be overlooked as an honorable and valuable attribute, partly due to practicality. It can be hard to determine if someone is humble. When researchers ask people to evaluate their humility, and they rate themselves a perfect five stars, is that really being humble? This contradiction of humility is why you may not hear of it as often as gratitude, compassion, and optimism among happiness science. Being humble is challenging to study and quantify.[188]

Courtesy of Marcia Merrins

Today I will reflect on being humble. Journal about three examples that show your humility on a routine basis. Name a few things you have done this week that you would consider humble. It has been shown that people that are more humble enjoy better physical and mental health.

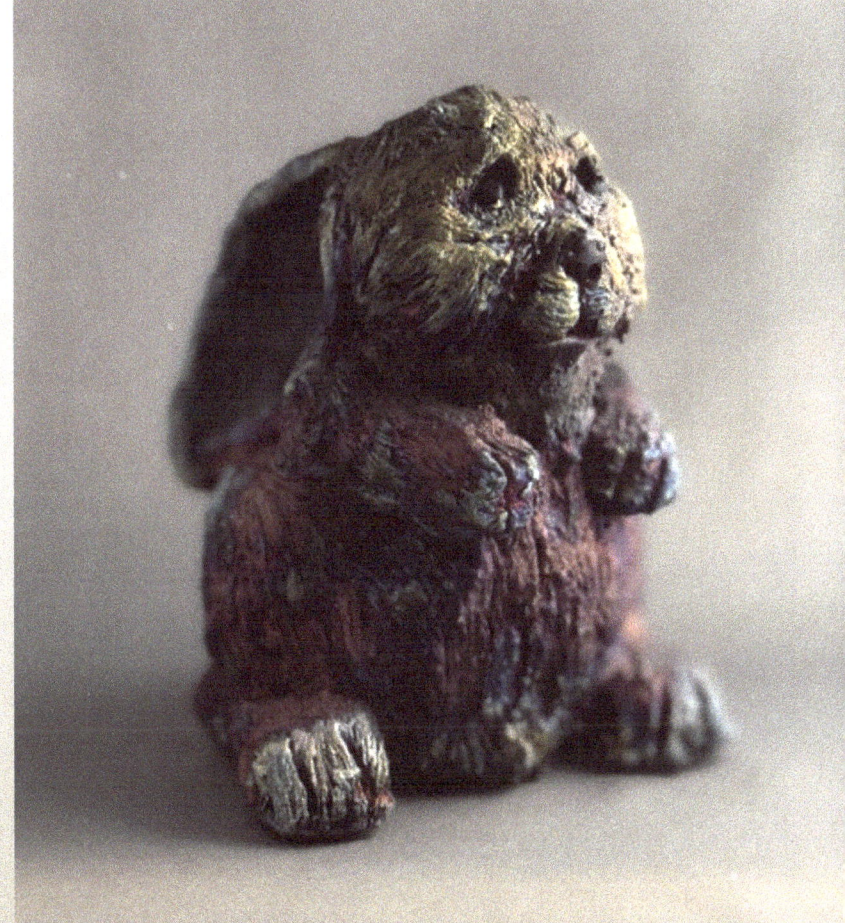

JUNE 26

Day 177

Feelings of Self-Doubt

Today, I didn't want to do anything. I feel exhausted from working hard and sleep deprivation from the course this country is on. I felt defeated and very discouraged. I didn't feel motivated and got nothing accomplished. I kept overthinking and had feelings of self-doubt. I wondered if anything I am doing is really worthwhile. Is my business sustainable? The stability in my life and my safety seem questionable. Is our country in complete chaos? I wonder if I should immigrate. I wonder how hard that would be. My mind was overloaded with these thoughts racing across my mind.[189]

Today I will calm my mind and let go of feelings of self-doubt. Consider how exhaustion, lack of sleep, and discouragement can bring a person down to the depth of despair. Journal about five things that have gone well for you over the past year and celebrate your successes. Turn on some upbeat music, distract from the negative stresses of overthinking and self-defeat. Go exercise, meditate, or practice some other self-care activity today. You don't have to feel defeated.

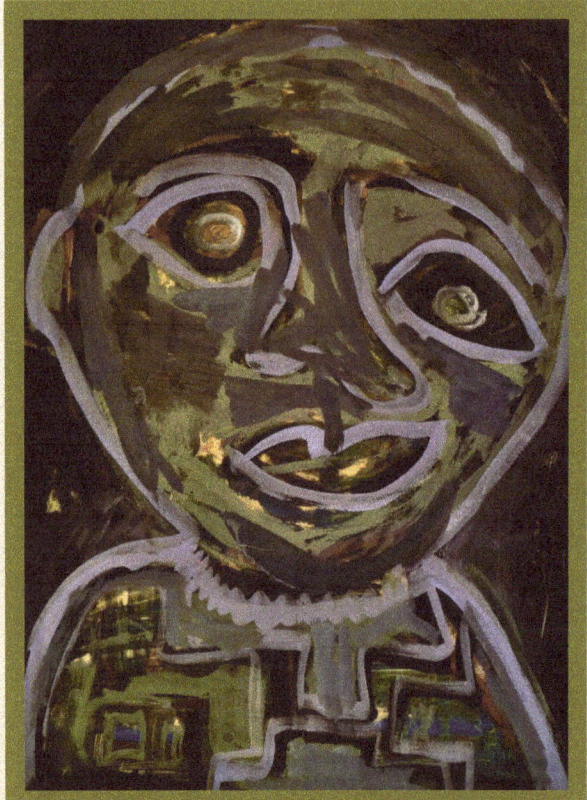

Courtesy of Robert John Holland

JUNE 27

Day 178

My Accomplishments

It's alright for me to share my accomplishments and successes – but I must do it authentically and in a humble way.[190]

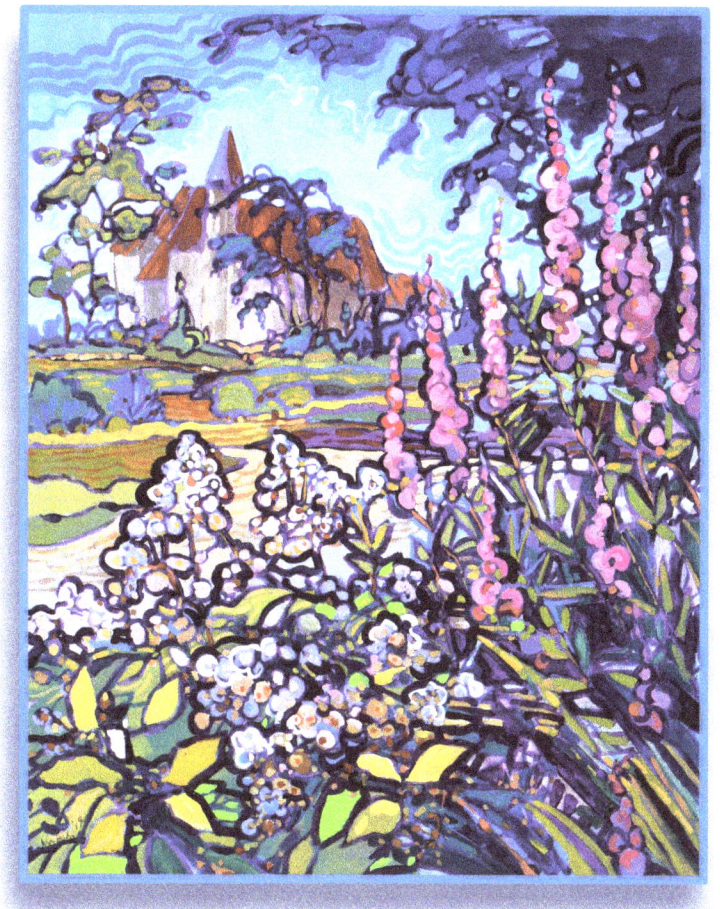

Courtesy of Judy Hodge

Today I will think about my accomplishments. What have you done so far in your life that make you the most proud? The top three things should roll right off your tongue. Knowing your accomplishments makes you self-aware of your value and allows you to feel proud. When you take notice of your accomplishments, you are acknowledging your authentic self. It's okay to share your successes. Journal about your three favorites, now.

JUNE 28
Day 179

Starting Small

I am noticing more lately that wonderful things often happen by starting small. We ought to actualize things in smaller steps. When starting small, we are most able to succeed.[191]

Today I will realize that everything doesn't have to be an enormous mountain. Small businesses are the staple of the American economy. Looking at the small steps in life can lead to bigger things. I can start small, and that's okay. When you start small, a day goes by, a week, then a month, and suddenly you have accomplished quite a bit. Journal about how you can focus on right now. What small steps can you start working towards today? Can you imagine the future bringing success by breaking ideas down into tiny pieces? If you start small, you can watch things grow big.

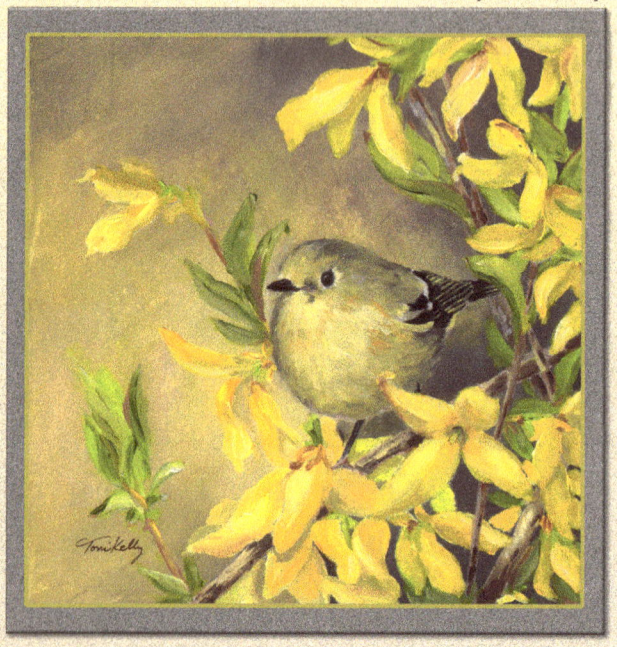

Courtesy of Toni Kelly

JUNE 29

Day 180

Thinking Big

Think about not how things really are, but what they could potentially be. There is so much value in visualizing by thinking big. Thinking big allows you to see what you can accomplish for your future. Don't be stuck in the present.[192]

Today I will think about something big that I would like to accomplish. Visualize it already being completed, and you're relaxing and relishing in the moment of completion, free of any stress or magical thinking. Can you think of two or three things you may have in mind? For instance, maybe you want to buy a new house, get a new job, or start a new relationship. Whatever it is, write your big thoughts down in your journal now.

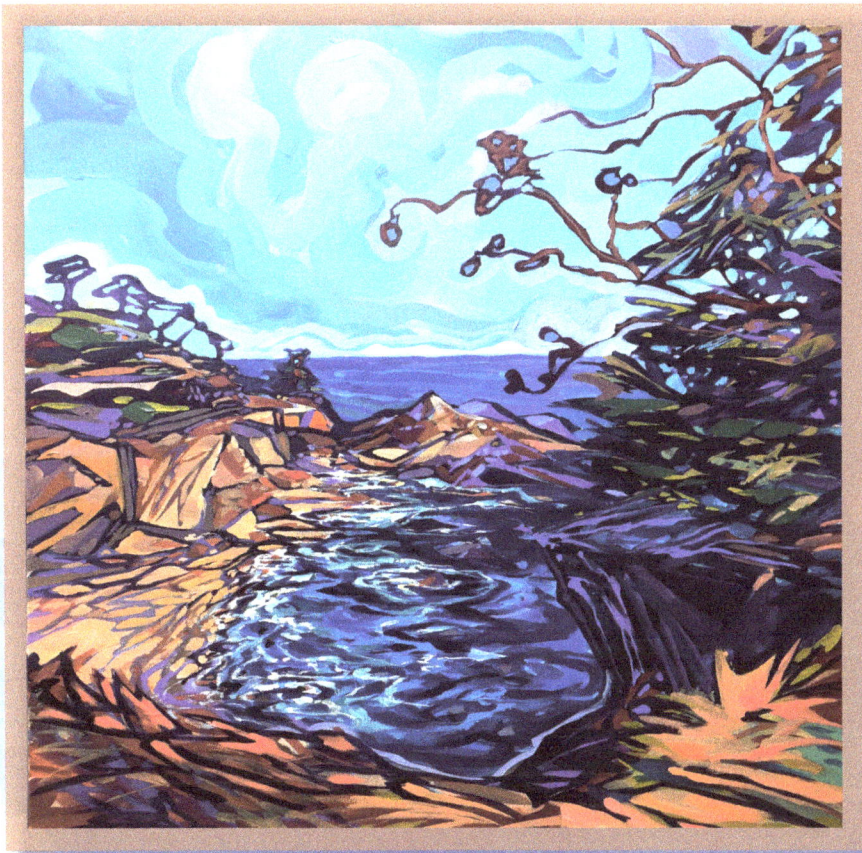

Courtesy of Judy Hodge

JUNE 30

Day 181

Workaholism

Like many addictions, work addiction can worsen with time until a person is willing to seek help. Workers might experience "burnout" by working themselves to a state of mental and physical exhaustion. This is a frequent outcome of work addiction. Burnout often leads to damaged relationships, extreme stress, and possibly even drug abuse. Without seeking treatment, someone with an addiction to work might distance themselves from their family and friends. Chronic stress may also result from continually working and can be harmful to physical health. Waiting longer to seek help with workaholism could permanently harm relationships.[193]

Today I will seriously consider getting some help if I am a workaholic. Life is not meant to be lived by being chained to your desk or tasks, constantly under stress. Assess your workload. You need to relax, enjoy, practice good self-care, and have a good work-life balance. Only you can control your work habits. Journal about times when you may have overworked yourself. What did you do to find relaxation? Were you able to seek help before becoming burned out? Find a support group if you cannot stop the urge to keep working.

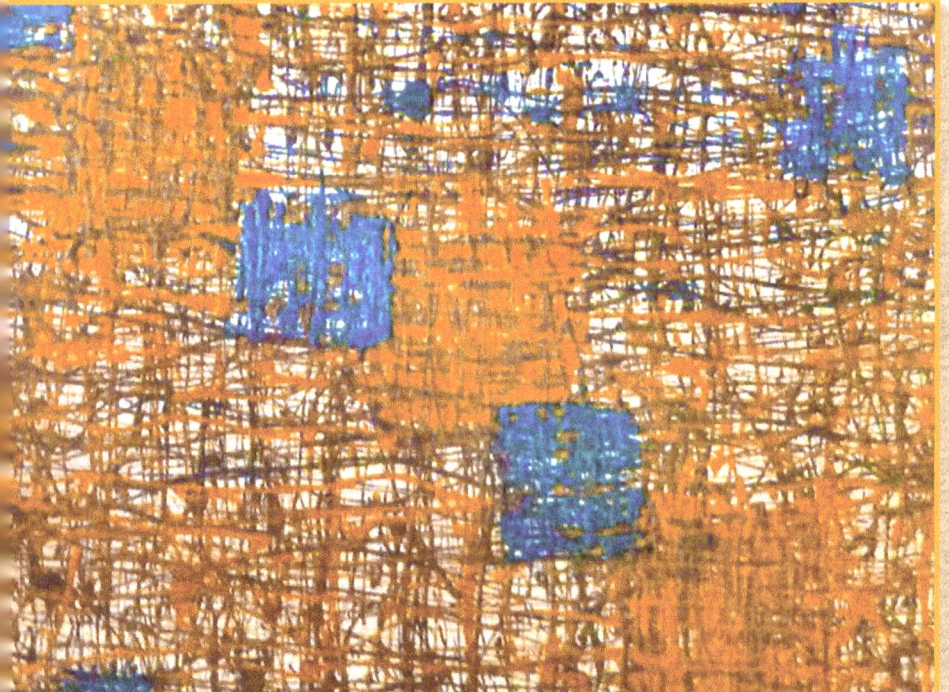

Courtesy of Aryn Grayson

References

[1] National Academy of Sciences. Taking Action Against Clinician Burnout: A Systems Approach to Professional Well-Being. National Academy of Medicine. Consensus Study Report. 2019 Oct. https://nam.edu/wp-content/uploads/2019/10/CR-report-hightlights-brief-final.pdf.. Accessed December 9, 2019.

[2] AMN Leadership Solutions. 2020 Healthcare Trends. AMN Healthcare. 2020. https://www.amnhealthcare.com/uploadedFiles/MainSite/Content/Campaigns/10-healthcare-trends-white-paper-2020.pdf.. Accessed April 14, 2020.

[3] National Academy of Sciences. Taking Action Against Clinician Burnout: A Systems Approach to Professional Well-Being. National Academy of Medicine. Consensus Study Report. 2019 Oct. https://nam.edu/wp-content/uploads/2019/10/CR-report-hightlights-brief-final.pdf.. Accessed December 9, 2019.

[99] Palmer Group. The Importance of Open Communication in the Workplace. Palmer Group: Employee Owned. 2020 Jan. https://thepalmergroup.com/blog/the-importance-of-open-communication-in-the-workplace/. Accessed February 1, 2020.

[100] Ruhmann J. 5 Ways to Celebrate Success with Your Team. Level Up Leadership. 2017 Dec. http://levelupleadership.com/5-ways-to-celebrate-success-with-your-team/. Accessed February 1, 2020.

[101] Dewhurst S. Burnout: A Hidden Enemy of Innovation and Well-Being in the Innovation Economy. Democrat & Chronicle. 2016 Aug. https://www.democratandchronicle.com/story/money/business/blogs/innovation/2016/08/03/burnout-a-hidden-enemy-of-innovation-and-well-being-in-the-innovation-economy/87995982/. Accessed February 1, 2020.

[102] Glenn C. Adaptability Equals Longevity. Thrive Global. 2019 Nov. https://thriveglobal.com/stories/adaptability-equals-longevity/. Accessed February 3, 2020.

[103] Mahajan G. What is Customer Value and How Can You Create It? Customer Think. 2016 Jan. https://customerthink.com/what-is-customer-value-and-how-can-you-create-it/. Accessed February 3, 2020.

[104] Jordan J, Watcha D, Cassella C, Kaji AH, Trivedi S. Impact of a Mentorship Program on Medical Student Burnout. Wiley Online Library. 2019 May; 3(3):218-225. https://onlinelibrary.wiley.com/doi/abs/10.1002/aet2.10354. Accessed February 3, 2020.

[105] Gallo A, Bernstein A, Torres N, Chow R. Sponsorship: Defining the Relationship. Harvard Business Review. 2019 Oct; 4(3). https://hbr.org/podcast/2019/10/sponsorship-defining-the-Relationship. Accessed February 3, 2020.

[106] Sanchez R. Sponsoring and Promoting Women and Minorites in Tech. Medium: Austin Startups. 2017 May. https://austinstartups.com/sponsoring-and-promoting-women-and-minorities-in-tech-43ff2364646. Accessed February 3, 2020.

[107] Meinert D. Emotional Intelligence is Key to Outstanding Leadership. SHRM. 2018 Feb. https://www.shrm.org/hr-today/news/hr-magazine/0318/pages/emotional-intelligence-is-key-to-outstanding-leadership.aspx. Accessed February 3, 2020.

[108] Gaither C. The Very Real Connections Between Job Burnout and Suicide. Clark Gaither. 2018 June. www.clarkgaither.com/the-very-real-connections-between-job-burnout-and-suicide/. Accessed February 3, 2020.

[109] Gordon-Mead W. Feeling More Irritable? This May Be the Reason. Thrive Global. 2019 July. https://thriveglobal.com/stories/feeling-more-irritable-this-may-be-the-reason/. Accessed February 3, 2020.

[110] Deschene L. 40 Ways to Create Piece of Mind. Tiny Buddha. 2017 Oct. https://tinybuddha.com/blog/40-ways-to-create-peace-of-mind/. Accessed February 3, 2020.

[111] Jones D. 5 Ground Rules for Workplace Friendships. The Balance Careers. 2019 June. https://www.thebalancecareers.com/workplace-friendship-rules-1917678. Accessed February 3, 2020.

[112] Rushton CH. To Restore Humanity in Health Care, Address Clinician Burnout. The Hastings Center. 2020 Jan. https://www.thehastingscenter.org/to-restore-humanity-in-health-care-address-clinician-burnout/. Accessed February 3, 2020.

[113] Fatima S. Better Ways to Shine at Work. SkillsYouNeed. https://www.skillsyouneed.com/rhubarb/shine-at-work.html. Accessed February 4, 2020.

[114] Perlo J, Swensen S, Kabcenell A, Landsman J, Feeley D. IHI Framework for Improving Joy in Work. Institute for Healthcare Improvement. 2017. http://www.ihi.org/resources/Pages/IHIWhitePapers/Framework-Improving-Joy-in-Work.aspx. Accessed February 4, 2020.

[115] Settembre J, Caprino K. 61% of Women Believe that Being Excluded at Work is a Form of Bullying. MarketWatch. 2018 Nov. https://www.marketwatch.com/story/61-of-women-believe-that-being-excluded-at-work-is-a-form-of-bullying-2018-11-14. Accessed February 4, 2020.

[116] OSHA. Workplace Violence OSHA Fact Sheet. U.S. Department of Labor: Occupational Safety and Health Administration. 2002. https://www.osha.gov/OshDoc/data_General_Facts/factsheet-workplace-violence.pdf. Accessed February 4, 2020.

[117] Vikings in Oslo. How to Build Greater Autonomy at Work. Timely Blog. 2019 July. https://memory.ai/timely-blog/how-to-build-greater-autonomy-at-work. Accessed February 4, 2020.

[118] Weisburg E. The Symptoms of Entrepreneurial Burnout: What You Should Look for to Avoid Burnout. Thrive Global. 2019 Nov. https://thriveglobal.com/stories/the-symptoms-of-entrepreneurial-burnout/. Accessed February 4, 2020.

[119] Matsudaira K. If You Want to Shine at Work, Do These 5 Things. Lifehack. 2014 May. https://www.lifehack.org/articles/work/you-want-shine-work-these-5-things.html. Accessed February 4, 2020.

[120] Boissy A. Why Resilience Training Isn't the Antidote for Burnout. Cleveland Clinic: Consult QD. 2017 Oct. https://consultqd.clevelandclinic.org/why-resilience-training-isnt-the-antidote-for-burnout/. Accessed February 5, 2020.

[121] Hoomans J. Avoiding Burnout: Renewal Requires More than Rest. The Leading Edge. 2014 Sep. https://go.roberts.edu/leadingedge/avoiding-burnout-renewal-requires-more-than-rest. Accessed February 5, 2020.

[122] Martinuzzi B. Why It's Important to Be Gracious Every Day. American Express: Business Trends and Insights. 2012 Dec. https://www.americanexpress.com/en-us/business/trends-and-insights/articles/top-10-ways-to-be-gracious/. Accessed February 5, 2020.

[123] Kaundart C. 5 Ways to Process Feedback at Work Without Triggering a Stress Response. Trello. 2019 Feb. https://blog.trello.com/process-feedback-at-work-stress. Accessed February 5, 2020.

[124] Halford S. 5 Steps for Giving Productive Feedback. Entrepreneur. 2011 Apr. https://www.entrepreneur.com/article/219437. Accessed February 7, 2020.

[125] Leong L. Seeking Approval and Being Competitive at Work is a Waste of Time. ABC Life. 2019 May. https://www.abc.net.au/life/seeking-approval-and-being-competitive-at-work-is-waste-of-time/11112778. Accessed February 7, 2020.

[126] Fisher M. Social Support Systems. Johns Hopkins Medicine. 2018 Aug. https://www.hopkinsmedicine.org/johns_hopkins_bayview/community_services/services/called_to_care/social_support_systems.html. Accessed February 7, 2020.

[127] Parton D. Dolly Parton Quotes (Author of Dolly). Goodreads. 2020. https://www.goodreads.com/author/quotes/144067.Dolly_Parton. Accessed February 7, 2020.

[128] Department of Labor. Enthusiasm and Attitude. Mastering Soft Skills for Workplace Success. 2020. https://www.dol.gov/odep/topics/youth/softskills/Enthusiasm.pdf. Accessed February 7, 2020.

[129] Street E. 5 Ways Successful People Overcome Major Obstacles. Learning Liftoff. 2015 Jan. https://www.learningliftoff.com/5-ways-successful-people-overcome-major-obstacles/. Accessed February 7, 2020.

[130] Siegler JE, Patel NN, Dine CJ. Prioritizing Paperwork Over Patient Care: Why Can't We Do Both? J Grad Med Educ. 2015 Mar; 7(1):16-18. https://www.ncbi.nlm.nih.gov/pmc/articles/PMC4507919/. Accessed February 7, 2020.

[131] Gaertner S. The Courage to Fail – Why It's Important to Embrace Negative Results. The Wiley Network. 2019 July. https://www.wiley.com/network/latest-content/the-courage-to-fail-why-it-s-important-to-embrace-negative-results. Accessed February 8, 2020.

[132] Myatt M. 10 Communication Secrets of Great Leaders. Forbes. 2012 Apr. https://www.forbes.com/sites/mikemyatt/2012/04/04/10-communication-secrets-of-great-leaders/#69cede922fe9. Accessed February 8, 2020.

[133]Bhasin K. 9 Surefire Ways to Destroy Employee Morale. American Express: Business Trends and Insights. 2017 Sep. https://www.americanexpress.com/en-us/business/trends-and-insights/articles/9-surefire-ways-to-destroy-employee-morale/. Accessed February 8, 2020.

[134]Connor S. Is Pessimism Really Bad for You? The Guardian. 2016 Nov. https://www.theguardian.com/society/2016/nov/20/is-pessimism-bad-for-you. Accessed February 8, 2020.

[135]Morin A. 3 Times Optimism Does You More Harm than Good. Business Insider. 2017 Nov. https://www.businessinsider.com/overly-optimistic-isnt-the-same-as-mentally-strong-2017-11. Accessed February 8, 2020.

[136]KWSM. How to Take on New Challenges at Work. Carter Law Firm: Labor & Class Action. 2015 Oct. http://carterlawfirm.net/how-to-take-on-new-challenges-at-work/. Accessed February 8, 2020.

[137]Galpin D, Maksymluk A, Whiteford A. Social Workers are Being Blamed for Their Own Stress and Burnout. The Guardian. 2019 July. https://www.theguardian.com/society/2019/jul/31/social-workers-stress-burnout-resilience. Accessed February 8, 2020.

[138]Torberg S. Importance of Taking a Vacation. Allina Health. 2017 June. https://www.allinahealth.org/healthysetgo/thrive/importance-of-taking-vacation. Accessed February 8, 2020.

[139]Mathews S. The Authentic Self: With a Capital "S". Psychology Today. 2018 Feb. https://www.psychologytoday.com/us/blog/traversing-the-inner-terrain/201802/the-authentic-self. Accessed February 8, 2020.

[140]Cronkleton E. How to Build Up Your Stamina. Healthline. 2017 Apr. https://www.healthline.com/health/fitness-exercise/how-to-increase-stamina. Accessed February 8, 2020.

[141]Herrick S. Why You Should Strive for Excellence at Work, Not Perfection. Cube Rules. 2019 Nov. https://cuberules.com/2019/11/08/strive-to-achieve-excellence/. Accessed February 9, 2020.

[142] Goyette K. Conquer Burnout with These 5 Ways to Cultivate Perseverance in Your Employees. Entrepreneur. 2018 Aug. https://www.entrepreneur.com/article/319248. Accessed February 9, 2020.

[143] Nauman E. Can Mindfulness Help Stop Health Worker Burnout? Greater Good Magazine. 2014 Mar. https://greatergood.berkeley.edu/article/item/can_mindfulness_help_stop_health_worker_burnout. Accessed February 9, 2020.

[144] Antonio T. 8 Powerful Benefits of Writing Things Down. Productive and Free. 2017 Feb. https://www.productiveandfree.com/blog/writing-things-down-benefits. Accessed February 9, 2020.

[145] Gambs J. What Does it Mean to be Socially Aware? Taylor & Francis Online. 2013 Sep; 19(2):51. https://www.tandfonline.com/doi/abs/10.1080/00094056.1942.10725688?journalCode=uced20&. Accessed February 9, 2020.

[146] Simon S. Mood and Burnout: The Connection and the Solution. Dynamic Chiropractic. 2013 Aug; 31(16). https://www.dynamicchiropractic.com/mpacms/dc/article.php?id=56604. Accessed February 10, 2020.

[147] Amado-Boccara I, Donnet D, Olie JP. The Concept of Mood in Psychology. Encephale: PubMed. 1993 Mar-Apr; 19(2):117-122. https://www.ncbi.nlm.nih.gov/pubmed/8275897. Accessed February 10, 2020.

[148] Brooks R, Hardy E, Hogg C. Thriving at Work: 6 Things Every Organisation Can Do to Support Mental Health. Peakon. 2019 May. https://peakon.com/us/blog/peakon/thriving-at-work/. Accessed February 10, 2020.

[149] Braithwate J. Changing How We Think About Healthcare Improvement. The BMJ. 2018 May. https://www.bmj.com/content/361/bmj.k2014. Accessed February 10, 2020.

[150] Caruthers C. Grounding 101: Why, How, and When to Do It. DOYOUYOGA. 2014 Sep. https://www.doyou.com/grounding-101-why-how-and-when-to-do-it/. Accessed February 10, 2020.

[151] Sheth S. Nadi Shodhana Pranayama: Alternate Nostril Breathing. SRMD Yoga. YouTube. 2018 Sep. http://www.youtube.com/watch?v=111qFpRqhIQ&t=266s. Accessed February 10, 2020.

[152] Seppälä E. Burnout: How to Take Care of Others Without Burning Out. Time. 2017 Aug. https://time.com/collection/guide-to-happiness/4886913/how-to-take-care-of-others-without-burning-out/. Accessed February 10, 2020.

[153] Khan F, Rasli A, Shehzad K, Yasir M, Malik F. Job Burnout and Professional Development Among Universities Academicians. Research Gate. 2014 Oct. https://www.researchgate.net/publication/268215186_Job_Burnout_and_Professional_Development_Among_Universities_Academicians. Accessed February 10, 2020.

[154] Anderson C. The Advantages of Employee Involvement in Decision Making. Small Business- Chron. 2019 Mar. https://smallbusiness.chron.com/advantages-employee-involvement-decision-making-18264.html. Accessed February 11, 2020.

[155] Ghapar A. How to Stay Realistically Optimistic. LeaderEconomics.com. 2017 Aug. https://leaderonomics.com/personal/stay-realistically-optimistic. Accessed February 11, 2020.

[156] Timer E. How to Effectively Communicate with your Boss. TheJobNetwork. 2018 July. https://www.thejobnetwork.com/effective-communication-with-your-boss/. Accessed February 11, 2020.

[157] Hall K. Self-Validation. Psychology Today. 2014 July. https://www.psychologytoday.com/us/blog/pieces-mind/201407/self-validation. Accessed February 11, 2020.

[158] Stainer MB. B is for Michael Bungay Stainer: Doing Great Work. The Positive Encourager. 2018 Feb. https://www.thepositiveencourager.global/michael-bungay-stanier-on-doing-great-work-2/. Accessed February 11, 2020.

[159] Becker J. The Helpful Guide to Living an Intentional Life. Becoming Minimalist. 2019 Sep. https://www.becomingminimalist.com/the-helpful-guide-to-living-an-intentional-life/. Accessed February 11, 2020.

[160]Martin. The Importance of Ideas. TheUniversityBlog. 2010 Apr. https://theuniversityblog.co.uk/ 2010/04/26/the-importance-of-ideas/. Accessed February 11, 2020.

[161]Stasiulionyte L. 10 Tips to Achieve Anything You Want in Life. SUCCESS. 2016 Aug. https://www.success.com/10-tips-to-achieve-anything-you-want-in-life/. Accessed February 11, 2020.

[162]Kaplan RS. Reaching Your Potential. Harvard Business Review. 2008 Jul/Aug. https://hbr.org/2008/07/reaching-your-potential. Accessed February 11, 2020.

[163]Nelson D. The Essence of Reiki. Reiki Infinite Healer: Level 1. 2011. https://www.reikiinfinitehealer.com/author/dave-nelson. Accessed February 11, 2020.

[164]Koenig R. How to Communicate About a Work Problem. U.S. News & World Report. 2018 May. https://money.usnews.com/money/careers/company-culture/articles/2018-05-09/how-to-communicate-about-a-work-problem. Accessed February 13, 2020.

[165]Langan-Riekhof M, Avanni AB, Janetti A. Sometimes the World Needs a Crisis: Turning Challenges into Opportunities. Brookings. 2017 Apr. https://www.brookings.edu/research/sometimes-the-world-needs-a-crisis-turning-challenges-into-opportunities/. Accessed February 13, 2020.

[166]Wenderoth MC. Do You Find Networking Stressful? Try Being a Connector Instead. Ascend: Harvard Business Review. 2019 July. https://hbrascend.org/topics/do-you-find-networking-stressful-try-being-a-connector-instead/?utm_source=twitter&utm_medium=social&utm_campaign=hbr. Accessed February 13, 2020.

[167]Chopra D. Becoming a Peacemaker. DailyOM. 2020. https://www.dailyom.com/cgibin/courses/courseoverview.cgi?cid=731&aff=0. Accessed February 13, 2020.

[168]Grant A. Frustrated at Work? That Might Just Lead to Your Next Breakthrough. The New York Times. 2019 Mar. https://www.nytimes.com/2019/03/08/smarter-living/frustrated-at-work-that-might-just-lead-to-your-next-breakthrough.html. Accessed February 19, 2020.

[169] Boynton B. "I Have to VENT!" as Nurses, Are We Letting Off Innocent Steam or Fueling Lateral Violence? Confident Voices in Healthcare. 2012 Feb. https://www.confidentvoices.com/2012/02/27/i-have-to-vent-as-nurses-are-we-letting-off-innocent-steam-or-fueling-lateral-violence/. Accessed February 19, 2020.

[170] BookBrowse. Well-knows Expressions: Nothing Ventured, Nothing Gained. BookBrowse.com. 1997-2020. https://www.bookbrowse.com/expressions/detail/index.cfm/expression_number/613/nothing-ventured-nothing-gained. Accessed February 19, 2020.

[171] Glynska M. Nothing Ventured, Nothing Gained: Is It Worth Taking Risks in Life? HuffPost. 2017 Dec. https://www.huffpost.com/entry/nothing-ventured-nothing-_b_11861514. Accessed February 19, 2020.

[172] Wyo.gov. Being Prepared. Wyoming Homeland Security. 2019. https://hls.wyo.gov/being-prepared. Accessed February 19, 2020.

[173] Penn State. Developing your Personal Career Strategy (PCS). Smeal MBA Career Services. 0AD. https://mba.smeal.psu.edu/careers-recruiting/career-preparation/personal_career_strategy.pdf. Accessed February 19, 2020.

[174] Ryan L. What If I Don't Want a Personal Brand? Forbes. 2016 June. https://www.forbes.com/sites/lizryan/2016/06/07/what-if-i-dont-want-a-personal-brand/#4dcc0c96399c. Accessed February 19, 2020.

[175] NHS. How to be happier. Nhs choices. https://www.nhs.uk/mental-health/self-help/tips-and-support/how-to-be-happier/. Published March 2, 2021. Accessed September 8, 2021.

[176] LaRocca B. Introduction to Social Awareness. Transforming Education. 2017 Apr. https://www.transformingeducation.org/introduction-to-social-awareness/. Accessed February 20, 2020.

[177] Executive Communicators Group. Presentation Skills: Voice. There's a Message in Your Voice. The Total Communicator. 2004; 2(3). http://totalcommunicator.com/vol2_3/voicemessage.html. Accessed February 21, 2020.

[178] Cross S. How to Voice Concerns Without Seeming Negative. AAT=Comment. 2019 Sep. https://www.aatcomment.org.uk/career/how-to-voice-concerns-without-seeming-negative-%EF%BB%BF/. Accessed February 21, 2020.

[179] Paracelsus Recovery. Burnout as an Underlying Cause of Addiction. Paracelsus Recovery. 2018 Dec. https://www.paracelsus-recovery.com/blog/burnout-as-an-underlying-cause-of-addiction/. Accessed February 21, 2020.

[180] Wilding M. 3 Types of Burnout, According to Psychologists (and Signs You're Headed for Trouble). Inc.com. 2018 Apr. https://www.inc.com/melody-wilding/3-types-of-burnout-according-to-psychologists-and-signs-youre-headed-for-trouble.html. Accessed February 21, 2020.

[181] Tepfenhart O. There's a Difference Between Being Honest & Being Mean. Bolde. 2016 Apr. https://www.bolde.com/theres-difference-honest-mean/. Accessed February 21, 2020.

[182] Huppert M. Employees Share What Gives Them a Sense of Belonging at Work. LinkedIn Talent Blog. 2017 Oct. https://business.linkedin.com/talent-solutions/blog/company-culture/2017/employees-share-what-gives-them-a-sense-of-belonging-at-work. Accessed February 24, 2020.

[183] Trump D. Quotes about Sticking to It. Quotes Gram. 0AD. https://quotesgram.com/quotes-about-sticking-to-it/. Accessed February 24, 2020.

[184] Levchuck C. If you Were Passed Over for a Promotion, Follow These Steps to Move Forward When you Didn't get to Move Up. Monster Contributor. 2020. https://www.monster.com/career-advice/article/promotion-denied-what-next-hot-jobs. Accessed February 24, 2020.

[185] Metlaine A, Sauvet F, Gomez-Merino D, et al. Sleep and Biological Parameters in Professional Burnout: A Psychophysiological Characterization. APA PsycNet. 2018 Jan. https://psycnet.apa.org/record/2018-16288-001. Accessed February 24, 2020.

[186] Horton AP. Here's When It's Worth Taking a Big Risk in Your Career. Fast Company. 2018 June. https://www.fastcompany.com/40590672/heres-when-its-worth-taking-a-big-risk-in-your-career. Accessed February 24, 2020.

[187] White DM. 5 Tips for Handling Workplace Drama. Psych Central. 2018 Oct. https://psychcentral.com /lib/5-tips-for-handling-workplace-drama/. Accessed February 24, 2020.

[188] Onderko P. Do These 6 Things to Be More Humble. SUCCESS. 2015 Nov. https://www.success.com/ do-these-6-things-to-be-more-humble/. Accessed February 24, 2020.

[189] Lala A. Feeling Discouraged and Defeated. Art of Happiness Institute. 2017 Apr. https://artofhappiness.institute/7-things-to-think-about-when-you-feel-discouraged-and-defeated/. Accessed February 26, 2020.

[190] Morin A. 7 Ways to Talk About Your Accomplishments Without Sounding Like A Braggart. Forbes. 2017 June. https://www.forbes.com/sites/amymorin/2017/01/29/7-ways-to-talk-about-your-accomplishments-without-sounding-like-a-braggart/#75371cf06fcc. Accessed February 26, 2020.

[191] Gascoigne J. The Habits of Successful People: They Start Small. Buffer Resources. 2016 Feb. https://buffer.com/resources/make-it-big-by-starting-small. Accessed February 26, 2020.

[192] Schwartz DJ. The Magic of Thinking Big Quotes by David J. Schwartz. Goodreads. 1987 Apr. https://www.goodreads.com/work/quotes/746042-the-magic-of-thinking-big. Accessed February 26, 2020.

[193] Tyler M, Legg TJ. Work Addiction: When Work Becomes an Addiction. Healthline. 2016 June. https://www.healthline.com/health/addiction/work. Accessed February 26, 2020.

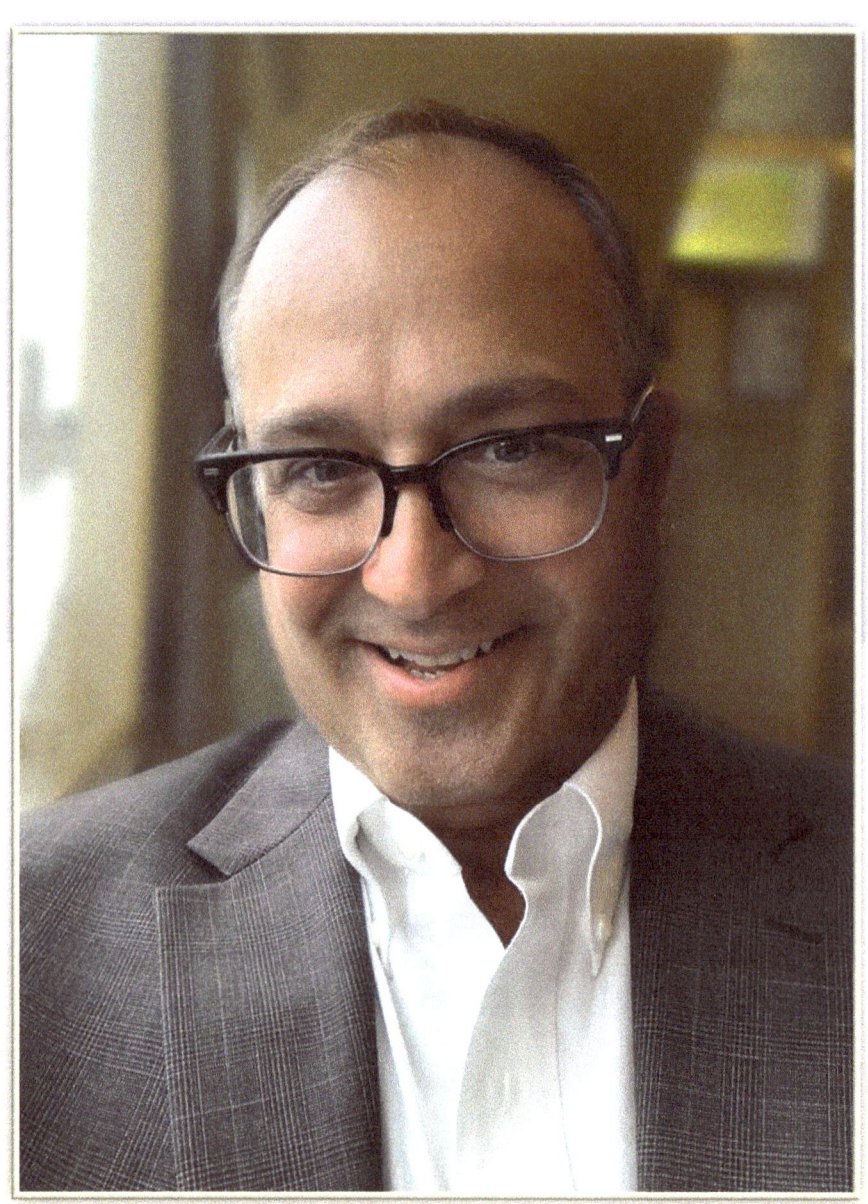

About the Author

Dr. Richard C. Scepura possesses strong credentials as a successful Nurse Executive. He is certified by American Nurses Credentialing Center as an Advanced Board-Certified Nurse Executive. He is also certified by the Nephrology Nursing Certification Commission as a Certified Dialysis Nurse. Richard has consulted and directed for *Seattle Children's Hospital, Steward Healthcare/St. Elizabeth's Medical Center* in Boston, MA, and managed for UNC Healthcare in Chapel Hill, NC. He began his career at *Beth Israel Deaconess Medical Center* (a Harvard teaching hospital) while living in the North End of Boston, MA, in the 1990s. He graduated from the University of Massachusetts with a double major Baccalaureate of Science in Psychology and Nursing. After several years as a staff RN, Richard began an exciting travel nurse career. He practiced in 14 U.S. states over a decade, working mostly in world-class magnet healthcare facilities across the nation serving different populations.

While working for UNC Hospitals, he attended Pfeiffer University in Research Triangle Park, NC, and received his joint degree, the MBA/MHA, Magna Cum Laude concentrating on Leadership and Change Management. His doctorate is in Nursing Practice (DNP) from Clarion and Edinboro Universities of Pennsylvania, graduating Summa Cum Laude. His doctoral project is titled, "*Intending to Stay - Retention, Burnout, Structural Empowerment and Dialysis Nursing: Integrating Kanter's Theory and the Refined Nurse Worklife Model*" and the abstract was selected for presentation at the American Nephrology Nursing Association National Symposium in May, 2021. He also published an article for the American Organization of Nurse Leaders in the *Nurse Leader* academic journal titled, "*The Challenges with Pre-Employment Testing and the Potential for Hiring Bias.*" He is a volunteer editorial board member for The American Journal of Management Science and Engineering as well as an editorial reviewer for MDPI: Nursing Reports Quarterly. Now, he brings to his colleagues, or any reader in need, in the most serious times of peril with Covid-19, the light-hearted thoughtful book that makes you "think," *The Healing Burnout Guide*.

Author's Note

A Special Thank You to the Artists- Without your talent, the self-reflection journals wouldn't be as purposeful. We appreciate your thoughtfulness and contributions in this great effort. We hope you enjoy the series and are sincerely pleased to promote your creations.

Artist Courtesy Credit List

Brown, Rachel	reb-brown@comcast.net
Chisholm, Jon	craigchism@twc.com
DelMonte, Barbara	barbaradelmonte2@gmail.com
Dunne, Kevin	kdunnek@gmail.com
Ensign, Nancy Nixon	nancynixonensign@gmail.com
French, Christine	christinefrench@me.com
Gonzalez, Maika	www.artmajeur.com/artedemaika/
Grayson, Aryn	nyra1266@gmail.com
Gutierrez, Susan	susanjgutierrez@outlook.com
Hodge, Judy	jhodge@urbanmindshare.com
Holland, Robert John	dotnbob@netsync.net
Julien, Marla	silversky26@hotmail.com
Kamperveen, Umberto	umberto@umbertokamperveenart.com
Kelly, Toni	toni@tonikellystudio.com
Lafferty, Ronnie	ronnielafferty60@gmail.com
Larson, Patti	pattilarsonphotos@outlook.com
Long, Charles Freedom	charlesfreedomlong@gmail.com
MacKay, Susan	smofny@stny.rr.com
Marquis, Eduardo Andres	eamt1966@gmail.com
Mattson, Jill	jillimattson@yahoo.com
Merrins, Marcia	mmerrins@netsync.net
Parker, Ann	anna242parker@yahoo.com
Probst, Linda	mikeandlindaprobst@yahoo.com
Rubin, Mara	rubinmaraci@hotmail.com
Samler, Rebecca	beckysamler1@gmail.com
Santi, Jill	jillswriting@hotmail.com
Schultz, Lisa	lschultz18102@gmail.com
Shank, Carrie	tothetopcj@gmail.com
Smith, Bill	Lorencsmith@twlakes.net
Spar Ki	sparki3114@icloud.com
Turner, Peter S.	psterlingtri@gmail.com

Contributors

Contributors:

Curator Nancy Nixon Ensign
Contributing Editor Tiffany Smith
Contributing Editor Jessica Olma
Graphic Designer Tom Olson & Pixel-Pencil Studio
Boutique Publisher Becky Norwood & Spotlight Publishing

The Artists of:

Barcelona, ES
Bennington, VT
Chautauqua County, NY
Erie County, NY
Erie County, PA
Gaios, GR
Manhattan, NY
Marathon, FL
Newport, RI
Toronto, CA

Peer Reviewers:

Dr. Jane Blystone, PhD
Dr. Meg Larson, DNP

Curator and Cover Background Art

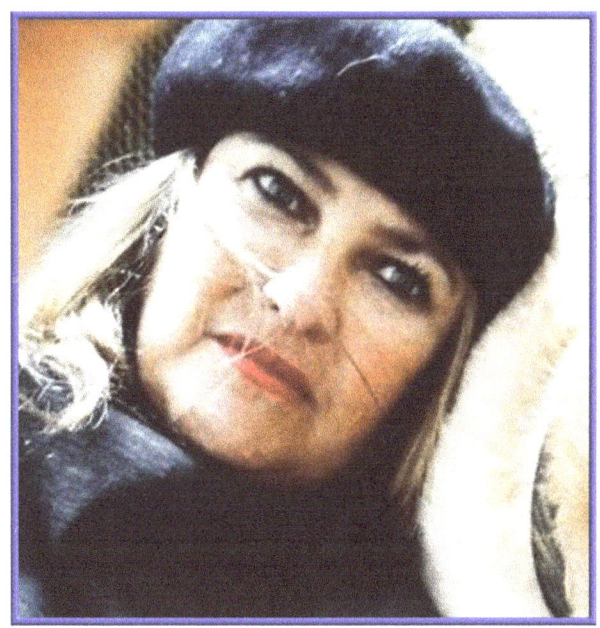

Nancy Nixon Ensign is a native Chautauqua County NY artist, third-generation maternal painter, and great-grandniece to impressionist *Edward Willis Redfield*. After graduating from *Rochester Institute of Technology* (RIT), she moved to Cleveland, OH, advancing her skills in ceramic and glass jewelry design while living at the *Hodge School Studios and Galleries*. Years later, Nancy moved to NYC to work as a set designer for *Victor Scenic* while also studying Byzantine Iconography at the *School of Sacred Arts*.

To escape winter, Nancy moved to Orlando, FL, and worked as a scenic artist for *Walt Disney World and Universal Studios*. Ten years later, she returned to Chautauqua County and was offered the position of *Patterson Library Octagon Gallery* Curator, installing well over 200 exhibitions. Currently, Nancy is Vice President and Exhibition Chair for the *North Shore Arts Alliance*, which she and seven other artists formed in 2008. Nancy and her husband, Jake, reside in Western New York, where she creates artwork in her home studio. *"I feel blessed and grateful to participate as curator, confidant, and friend to Richard."*

Contributing Editor

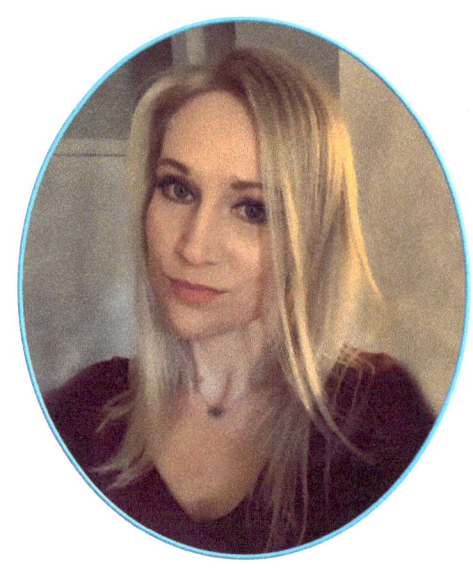

Tiffany Lynn Smith is a native of *Chautauqua County, NY*. After graduating from *Jamestown Community College* with an associate degree in Business Administration, she moved to Tempe, AZ, to continue her education at *Arizona State University (ASU)*. There, Tiffany studied and graduated with a BA in English Literature with a focus on Business and Professional Writing/Editing. In Arizona, she worked as a technical writer for Kizen Group, an ASU eSeed Venture.

Tiffany then moved to Charlotte, NC, where she currently resides. She has held management positions in both the service industry and retail, most recently for *Michael Kors*. She now works as an office administrator/medical assistant for *Lake Norman Integrative Wellness*. Tiffany is very passionate about technical writing and provides contractual editing services.

Contributing Editor

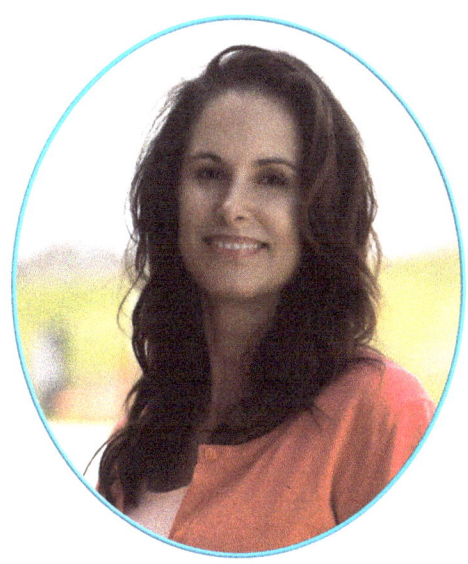

Jessica Olma is a writer and editor. Originally from Vancouver, BC, Canada, she obtained dual citizenship in the US and moved throughout the country, settling in North Coventry, PA, where she attended college at Temple University's Elkins Park Art Campus. In 2014, after raising her family, she attended Colorado Technical University to pursue her passion for writing and editing. Jessica established *Scribe Syndicate* in Charlotte, NC, to offer writing and editing services to various clients who publish information in print and online. As the business grew, she moved to Denver, CO, and collaborates nationally on digital marketing projects. Jessica works closely with publishers, authors, web designers, marketing consultants, and business owners to write and edit eBooks, web page copy, blog articles, white papers, and more. She ensures her clients are seen as experts in their field who provide high-quality information and education to the public and consumers. She is honored to be part of Dr. Richard Scepura's book, *The Healing Burnout Guide*.

Graphic Designer

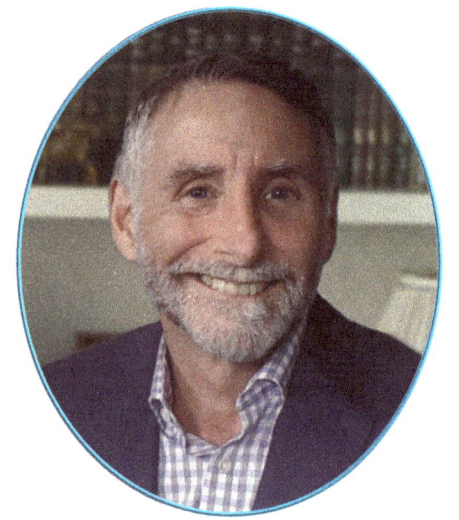

Tom Olson is the founder of Pixel-Pencil Studio, a graphic design agency in Rye, NY specializing in publications. With more than 20 years of Manhattan agency experience, Tom places the highest priority on superior client service, creativity and attention to detail.

https://PixelPencilStudio.com

Publisher

International Bestselling author, speaker, and book publishing expert, **Becky Norwood** is CEO of Spotlight Publishing™. Recognizing that writing and publishing a book is only the beginning of an author's journey, she encourages the authors she works with to implement sensible marketing to gain exposure for their work.

Through her Author Studio TV Show, countless listeners have heard her interviews of both authors and experts offering sage advice. Additionally, she offers a catalog of services supporting emerging and established authors, working with joint venture partners well-versed in their fields.

Becky believes that a well-told story is a gateway for growth, sharing, and a way to unite humanity. She advocates for the positive that comes from sharing our creative genius and impacting our world in positive ways.

https://SpotlightPublishing.Pro

SEASON TWO

Competent

APRIL 1

Day 91

Open Communication

APRIL 2

Day 92

Celebrating Success

APRIL 3

Day 93

Innovation

APRIL 4

Day 94

Adaptability

APRIL 5

Day 95

Creating Value

APRIL 6

Day 96

Mentorship

APRIL 7

Day 97

Sponsorship

APRIL 8

Day 98

Emotional Intelligence

APRIL 9

Day 99

Burnout and Suicide

APRIL 10

Day 100

Feeling Irritable

APRIL 11

Day 101

Regaining Peace

APRIL 12

Day 102

Friendship at Work

APRIL 13

Day 103

Humanity

APRIL 14

Day 104

Soft Skills

APRIL 15

Day 105

Finding Joy through Work

APRIL 16
Day 106

Exclusion from Decision-Making

APRIL 17

Day 107

Violence in the Workplace

APRIL 18

Day 108

Need for Greater Autonomy

APRIL 19

Day 109

Entrepreneurship

APRIL 20

Day 110

Shining at Work

APRIL 21

Day 111

Resilience

APRIL 22

Day 112

Renewal

APRIL 23

Day 113

Being Gracious

APRIL 24

Day 114

Receiving Feedback

APRIL 25

Day 115

Giving Feedback

APRIL 26

Day 116

Competitiveness

APRIL 27

Day 117

Support Systems

APRIL 28

Day 118

Dream More

APRIL 29

Day 119

Enthusiasm at Work

APRIL 30

Day 120

Overcoming Obstacles

MAY 1

Day 122

Documentation Demand

MAY 2

Day 123

Courage to Fail

MAY 3

Day 124

Communicating from the Heart

MAY 4

Day 125

Morale

MAY 5

Day 126

Pessimism

MAY 6

Day 127

Overly Optimistic

MAY 7

Day 128

New Challenges

MAY 8

Day 129

Blame

MAY 9

Day 130

Taking a Vacation

MAY 10

Day 131

Authentic Self

MAY 11

Day 132

Stamina

MAY 12

Day 133

Excellence

MAY 13

Day 134

Perserverance

MAY 14

Day 135

Being Mindful

MAY 15

Day 136

Write it Down

MAY 16

Day 137

Socially Aware

MAY 17

Day 138

Mood

MAY 18

Day 139

Thriving

MAY 19

Day 140

Constant Changes

MAY 20

Day 141

Firmly Grounded

MAY 21

Day 142

Serving Others

MAY 22

Day 143

Professional Development

MAY 23
Day 144

Involvement in Decision-making

MAY 24 Day 145

Realistic Optimism

MAY 25

Day 146

Talking with your Boss

MAY 26

Day 147

Validate Yourself

MAY 27

Day 148

Doing Great Work

MAY 28

Day 149

Being Intentional

MAY 29

Day 149

My Ideas

MAY 30

Day 150

Be Curious

MAY 31

Day 151

My Full Potential

JUNE 1

Day 152

Being Thankful

JUNE 2

Day 153

Expressing Concerns

JUNE 3

Day 154

Challenges Into Opportunities

JUNE 4

Day 155

Networking

JUNE 5

Day 156

Making Peace

JUNE 6

Day 157

Frustration

JUNE 7

Day 158

Venting

JUNE 8
Day 159

Nothing Ventured, Nothing Gained

JUNE 9

Day 160

Being Prepared

JUNE 10

Day 161

Develop Your Own Career Strategy

JUNE 11

Day 162

Your Brand

JUNE 12 Day 163

Feel Good

JUNE 13

Day 164

Social Awareness

JUNE 14 *Day 165*

Tone, Volume, and Cadence

JUNE 15

Day 166

Legitimate Concerns

JUNE 16

Day 167

Addictions

JUNE 17

Day 168

Types of Burnout

JUNE 18

Day 169

Being Truthful, Not Hurtful

JUNE 19

Day 170

Belonging

JUNE 20

Day 171

Sticking With It

JUNE 21

Day 172

Being Denied Opportunities

JUNE 22 *Day 173*

My Sleep Pattern

JUNE 23

Taking Risks

Day 174

JUNE 24

Day 175

Unnecessary Drama

JUNE 25

Day 176

Being Humble

JUNE 26 — Day 177

Feelings of Self-Doubt

JUNE 27

Day 178

My Accomplishments

JUNE 28

Day 179

Starting Small

JUNE 29

Day 180

Thinking Big

JUNE 30

Day 181

Workaholism

CPSIA information can be obtained
at www.ICGtesting.com
Printed in the USA
BVHW011115200423
662721BV00019B/689